DEVELOPMENT AND THE PROBLEMS OF VILLAGE NUTRITION

Development and the Problems of Village Nutrition

SUE SCHOFIELD

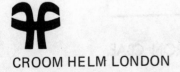

CROOM HELM LONDON

in association with

THE INSTITUTE OF DEVELOPMENT STUDIES, SUSSEX

© 1979 Institute of Development Studies
Croom Helm Ltd, 2–10 St John's Road, London SW11

British Library Cataloguing in Publication Data

Schofield, Sue
  Development and the problems of village nutrition.
  1. Underdeveloped areas – Nutrition
  2. Underdeveloped areas – Village communities
  I. Title   II. Institute of Development Studies
  641.1'09172'4   TX357

  ISBN 0–85664–836–1

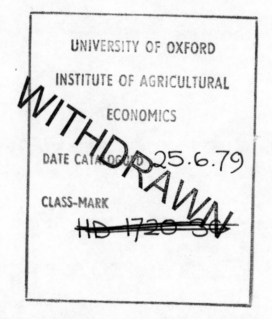

Printed in Great Britain by offset lithography by
Billing & Sons Ltd, Guildford, London and Worcester

CONTENTS

CONTENTS

TABLES

Tables

ACKNOWLEDGEMENTS

The research on which this book is based was conducted as part of the Village Studies Programme under the guidance of Professor Michael Lipton. I would like to thank him for giving me the opportunity to work in such an interesting and important field and for all the help and assistance he has given me throughout the project and in the writing of this book. Other members of the VSP team who helped me with the statistical analysis are Biblap Dasgupta and Roy Laishley. I would like to thank them and also the Freedom From Hunger Campaign Committee who financed this research and the Institute of Development Studies which provided funding for its completion.

1 INTRODUCTION

The words 'famine' or 'mass starvation' are emotional terms which motivate intermittent action in the form of international aid and national help. But famines are the tip of the iceberg which emerges every so often in response to unusually drastic conditions. Underneath this tip is a continual process of malnourishing which is both a consequence of economic conditions in less developed countries and a contributory factor. Malnutrition in its moderate or mild forms is not as obvious as starvation but it constitutes a problem of immense proportions even in countries which are beginning to be self-sufficient in cereal grain production for calculated levels of current nutrition.

There is a general lack of reliable and comparable data on the incidence of nutritional deficiencies throughout the less developed world. Under-recording, especially of marginal cases, is the main problem. Investigations are restricted to small, unrepresentative samples and special groups; methods of data collection are variable and of poor quality; results are expressed in different ways and it is difficult to attach nutritional deficiency 'labels' to some symptoms. Even so, this evidence shows that in less developed countries, two-thirds of pre-school children suffer from malnutrition; between 0.2 and 1.6 per cent of children under 5 years of age are suffering from kwashiorkor (protein deficiency) and these are only the registered cases; its real incidence may be six or eight times higher (Bengoa, 1973, p. 107). Marasmus (protein and calorie deficiency) is even more common and present in 1.2 to 6.8 per cent of the pre-school population although its incidence may be on the increase in countries such as Chile where early weaning is fast becoming established. Of the other deficiencies, anaemia is the cause of most maternal deaths in India (Gopalan, 1969) where its incidence in pregnant women, of whom there are at least 20 million at any given time, is especially high. In Africa, 6–17 per cent of men, 15–50 per cent of women and 30–60 per cent of children under 15 are anaemic (FAO, 1970). Symptoms of Vitamin A deficiency are also highly prevalent in the less developed world and the cause of most cases of preventable blindness. The incidence of all other deficiency diseases (rickets, scurvy, etc.) varies from country to country.

Given this magnitude of malnutrition, and the belief that an adequate diet is the basic right of all human beings independent of class and income, we scarcely need justify the need for nutrition policies and intervention programmes. Nutrition is but one component of human welfare, enhancement of which should be the prior and major concern of all government efforts at economic development. As such, it has a legitimate claim on public resources, expenditure and efforts. We also

11

need to consider that malnutrition is an impediment to national growth because it reduces work output and life expectancy; it is one of the causes of high infant mortality and it impairs mental development and therefore reduces the effectiveness of investments in education.

Poverty is the underlying cause of most malnutrition: those who are malnourished are the bottom 30 per cent of the population, with low incomes and little political motivation or support. The majority of low-income families are located in rural areas where the most acute nutritional problems are found now and will be located in the future except when as famine victims they flock to city centres to seek jobs and food. The poor spend a very high proportion — often as much as 80 per cent — of their total income on food, and cross-section survey data show that a large part of additions to their income are also spent on foods and usually on cereals and food grains with high amounts of calories and proteins per penny than on more expensive foods. Thus there can be no doubt that increases in real income will lead to dietary improvements for most people. However, in most less developed countries, incomes are unequally distributed and economic growth is rarely reflected in income increments for the poor. Standards of living are not improving at substantial rates and even in countries where the general level of national output has risen and national incomes increased, there has been no parallel eradication of poverty.

Thus economic growth alone cannot be expected to improve nutritional conditions unless governments undertake policies to redistribute incomes or assets, to steer income growth to the poor or to restructure food supplies. Programmes could include the redistribution of land, price reductions in specific purchases for certain income groups, rationing, shifts in wages, rents or prices or improving human capital through education and health schemes. Such broad measures involve social and economic changes of a vast political nature, needing support from the electorate. These are long-term solutions but meanwhile the poor must suffer and remain hungry. Marginal intervention measures or short-term nutrition programmes are the only viable alternative to creating fuller employment or raising the income of the most vulnerable groups. Since these groups are too poor to attract private enterprise, government intervention in this field is also inevitable and generally takes one or both of two alternative forms.

The first approach identifies the cause of nutritional problems — whether regional, local or within villages — as one of an inadequate national supply of food. In comparison, nutritionists see the problem in terms of nutrient deficiencies of vulnerable groups, communities and individuals. Compared with nutrition, food is an obviously tangible asset: available supplies can be measured; future supplies projected; costs estimated and national food accounts constructed. Nutrition on the other hand is a much vaguer term meaning little'to planners in the way of measurable assets. It is not surprising therefore that governments concern themselves with food and agricultural policies (whose main component is often to increase food consumption) and assume that these will naturally incorporate and provide solutions to nutritional problems. Predicting fluctuations in food supplies is obviously valuable for timing emergency action so that famines are given priority by governments and international organisations but emergency famine relief is too expensive to be on-going and may not even be dealing with the heart of the matter if the predictions are wrong. Also, those most in need of more food still have no guarantee of being able to afford the increased supplies of food on the market.

Therefore the second avenue of approach is to implement wide reaching, obvious, low-cost solutions, at the macro level, which treat nutritional deficiencies as a major epidemic equivalent to malaria or smallpox. 'Blanket' child feeding programmes which have a wide market, fulfil nutritional needs and meet commercial interests are but one example: fortification programmes are another. Blanket programmes reach selected groups by mass coverage of the entire populace but are very inefficient in achieving their objectives. If 30 per cent of the populace requires nutrition intervention, it is prohibitively costly to cover the whole population. Even then, the programme may only reach a small proportion of the target group.

What we hope to show is that broad, indiscriminate programmes which provide dispersed coverage are better replaced by more selective programmes instigated at the community level on the basis of strategic needs, i.e. target programmes. These still imply mass organisation and suffer from problems of co-ordination and administration but they are usually short-term interventions which are aimed solely at the selected group. They have clearer objectives, are controllable and more useful if resources are limited. Planning at macro level can obviously not be done away with but 'macro nutrition' would benefit from the decentralisation of planning processes to provide more active power at the local or micro level which is the individual and his localised community.

This book is concerned with the development of micro-level approaches (and one in particular) to nutrition problem identification since we believe that 'the process of malnourishing' (Knutsson, 1973, p. 31) can only really be examined, analysed and understood at the micro level where the whole range of factors affecting nutrition are displayed and individual, community and regional problems can be diagnosed to provide the basis for more meaningful action and plans. After all, nutrition is only one component of national economic development but it is an over-ridingly important part of the lives of poor villagers. Micro-level nutrition data provide information on diet patterns, nutritional status, food habits and on any other factors affecting or determining the type and extent of malnutrition. Successful micro-level action has two dimensions: firstly it helps to identify nutritional problems by region, ecological zone, village community or intra-village group and secondly the nature and causal determinants of the nutrition problem will be evaluated and the need for nutrition interventions assessed and measured against the need for other types of action.

Since a very high proportion of the population of less developed countries reside in rural areas and, to a large and known extent, in small, usually self-contained, defined, residential and land holding units called villages, we have taken, for our purposes, the individual as the villager and his community as the village. The village oriented approach to micro-level nutrition problems was initiated as a new approach to the study of development problems by the Village Studies Programme (VSP) at the Institute of Development Studies (IDS), University of Sussex. This programme was initiated in 1969. Since then, team members from the disciplines of anthropology, economics, history and geography have been conducting research under the guidance of Professor Michael Lipton. This programme has been generously financed by the Social Science Research Council (SSRC), the Ministry of Overseas Development (ODM), the International Labour Organisation of the World Employment Programme (ILO), the United Kingdom Branch of the Freedom From Hunger Campaign Committee (FFHCC) and the IDS.

In this book, the micro-level approach to nutrition problem identification is discussed in chapter 2 with particular reference to the village identification of nutrition problems adopted by the VSP. We are not concerned with programme selection or the development of methods and procedures for evaluating and selecting interventions. What we are concerned with are methods for collecting nutrition data and measuring nutritional status and methods or approaches for identifying types of nutritional problem at the micro level. This study focuses on all these problems and relies for its authenticity on second hand, micro-level data obtained from less developed countries all over the world. These data and methods of data collection are included in chapters 3 and 4 as a guide to planners, nutritionists and field workers. Types of data available by source are discussed so that planners know where to look for village specific nutrition data before instigating more data collecting surveys. The data and methods of collection are evaluated and their limitations discussed in order to acquaint future users with its quality and future data collectors with the sort of information that would be more useful to collect. Nutritional problems by type of village and within villages are discussed in chapters 5 and 6 and in chapter 7 we investigate problems of programme implementation at the local level.

2 APPROACHES TO THE IDENTIFICATION OF NUTRITION PROBLEMS AT THE MICRO LEVEL

Although accepted methods of planning exist in other fields of development, food and nutrition planning is still limited by the inadequacy of its conceptual approach. The stages in nutrition planning are not always sequential, clear cut or well ordered. The absence of an overall framework means that objectives are unclear and projects get accepted through the pressures of individuals and research institutes rather than through an ordered planning process which assesses needs and implements programmes to meet them.

The first stage in the planning sequence should be to identify the malnourished groups, determine why they are malnourished, what the nutritional deficiencies are and their severity and trends. The second step is the identification and costing of alternative programmes relevant to the needs of the malnourished. The programme is then selected, implemented, and eventual feedback enables evaluation of its success.

Problem Identification

Problem identification enables the planner to pinpoint the need, identify the type and cause of nutritional deficiencies, locate the population groups which are affected and measure the severity of the malnutrition. To assess the problem, nutritionists largely employ nutritional parameters and provide data on food expenditure, food production in relation to estimated population requirements, data on the incidence of types of deficiency disease, data on food and nutrient consumption and information on the physical status of the target group. Descriptive studies predominate: in India there are scores of studies measuring the number of persons below a stated caloric norm, but very few that link such undernutrition to the social or economic status of the family. Such research is functionless since 'to know how many people are short of nutrients and by how much is operationally meaningless unless one also knows who they are, and why they are undernourished' (Joy, 1973b, p. 5) and at what cost we can help.

Planners typically identify population groups as malnourished on the basis of age and physiological status. Traditionally, the 'vulnerable' groups are pre-school children, pregnant women and lactating mothers but this classification is unsatisfactory since we cannot assume for example that all pre-school children are suffering from protein calorie malnutrition; it may only be those in certain income groups, ecological zones or types of family who are really deprived of proteins and calories. In practice, other groups not usually identified as vulnerable may be worse off in certain situations, which indicates that new classifications of the malnourished population are required.

The classificatory approach to the identification of malnourished groups is gradually being accepted by planners. However, there are very few methods of classification available and these need to be more rigorously defined before they can be usefully applied. Here we concentrate on those which have received some recognition (functional and ecological classification, typical profiles and community diagnoses) and introduce another method of classification, by village type, which was adopted by the Village Studies Programme to provide solutions to problems of rural development in general, but also including nutrition.

Functional Classification
This method is described by Joy (1973b) who maintains that within any country, the primary nutritional classification is regional, based on the administrative structures. The identification of ecological sub-zones is next; followed by the classification of population sub-groups by economic status; the identification of demographic categories within these sub-groups by age and sex characteristics and then by deficiency pattern (chronic, seasonal or occasional) and type of nutrient deficiency or problem. These divisions will of course vary between countries. One country might be divisible into three administrative zones, each sub-divided into three ecological sub-zones (urban, rural accessible and rural inaccessible) and further subdivided by cropping areas and type of farming, etc. This will differ from another country with four administrative zones and even more ecological sub-zones. Eventually, however, functional classification needs to be quantified so that patterns of nutrient intake, height/weight ratios and morbidity/mortality data can be correlated with type of ecological zone and geographical location.

Ecological Classification
Nutritional differences between ecological zones have long been identified (Jelliffe, 1960) but not studied in depth or classified. Such studies are more common in Africa than any other less developed country. Diets are usually compared by type of food staple characteristic of the ecological zone (e.g. sorghum and millet based diets are compared with yam diets by Nicol, 1959). Exceptions are Cros's (1967) interesting study which compares the diets of Senegalese Forest and Savannah villages.

Ecological descriptions are usually brief and often based on superficial observations rather than in-depth studies. Villages are compared where conditions are 'favourable' or 'unfavourable' (Oomen, 1958) or differences in diet attributed to the fact that the population density is less and hunting activities more common in one village than another (Bailey, 1963). McKay's (1970) Malayan Longhouse survey is rather more detailed while there are other studies (Tan *et al.,* 1970) which concentrate on socio-cultural differences. Tan concluded that it is essential to adapt applied nutrition programmes to suit the local situation (Tan, 1970, pp. 97–8) and it is conclusions like these which should become more common with improved micro-level approaches.

Case Studies and Typical Profiles

Case studies are one of the primary methodological tools of intensive anthropological surveys in small communities. They are used in two ways:

(a) anthropologists pool their observations and classify forms of structural relationships and systems, citing cases to show how these systems 'work', or
(b) they describe case studies and extract the rule of custom or social relationship (Gluckman, 1967).

Recently, however, instead of remaining in the fieldworker's notebooks or being used as examples, case studies have been incorporated into analytical descriptions as part of the analysis to show changes over time (e.g. in social relations). They have also been quantified.

Typical profiles are detailed case studies of population sub-groups within a statistical frame. They have been identified in African communities by Jelliffe (1972b); discussed in terms of the rural subsistence community, the changing rural economy and the urban situation by Knutsson (1972) and four population groups which 'typify profiles found in many parts of the world' have been isolated by Berg (1973, p. 241). These include non-monetised subsistence groups; low income, partially monetised small farmers; low income, landless agricultural labourers and low income, urban migrants.

Ideally, profiles are characterised by a series of variables which define and determine their nutritional status (Berg and Muscat, 1973). Some of these variables are not quantifiable and not easy to identify and as yet there are no fixed rules for selecting relevant ones. Therefore, 'research will be necessary to provide the variables needed, to quantify qualitative variables, and to trace their inter-dependencies' (Ginor, 1973, p. 280). We must identify variables which are the main causes of malnutrition and those that can be most easily and successfully addressed by development programmes. Ideally, 'key' variables (e.g. income or size of landholding) have a greater effect on nutrition than others (e.g. absence of sanitation) meaning that redistribution of income or land would result in more or better nutritional improvements than programmes improving sanitation. The variables selected will differ for profiles of infant malnutrition in a rural cash crop zone, a health profile of adolescents in peri-urban settlements where incomes are low or a community profile in a desert zone. Ideally, profiles should 'serve as a kind of litmus paper against which any of the standard nutrition intervention programs can be tested' (Berg and Muscat, 1973, p. 260). As such, any difficulties in defining typical profiles are compensated for by the insights they provide into the causes of malnutrition and the data they supply for choosing between or combining programme alternatives.

Community Diagnoses

An alternative causal approach is community diagnosis which involves the identification of the nutritional problems within any group of people living and acting as a community. According to Dwarakinath (1967, p. 3) a community consists of individuals and groups interacting in a unit having a natural environment. Even so, communities are often difficult to identify as they vary from dispersed, isolated groups living in a defined area to cohesive but small groups existing within a larger social framework such as a village.

However, if the community is an easily identifiable administrative unit with a coherent structure, it can easily form the basis for a community diagnosis of malnutrition which should include the nature and extent of the problem, groups involved and the causes (Jelliffe, 1972b, p. 126). Such a diagnosis requires 'intensive, broad spectrum field research on malnutrition, in the many different types of local communities where people face the problems' (Knutsson, 1973, pp. 29–30). Only in this way can we determine the extent and causes of malnutrition. Some of these will be easy to find (bad roads or poor rainfall) but other information can only be acquired through careful and select questioning.

Village Typologies (The Village Studies Programme)

One problem basic to nutrition problem identification is that target groups traditionally identified as malnourished do not always fall within structured, administrative units useful for effective programme implementation. Communities are sometimes amorphous groups which are difficult to identify, while typical profiles may overlap administrative units. An alternative unit is the village. Nutritional problems can be identified by *types* of village, and within villages several profiles may be definable which can be reached far more effectively simply because the village is a primary administrative unit.

The village therefore became the primary focus of comparative research conducted by the Village Studies Programme (VSP). Our 'model' hypothesis with which we began the project was that differ-

ences among types of village explain the varying success of different
sorts of development efforts. The type of village – as indicated by a
few measures of its ecological, demographic and socio-economic
structure – largely determines the decisions of villagers in a less developed country and thus differences in rural behaviour and response.

The most obvious question to ask of the VSP is 'why villages?'; what
is so special about villages in less developed countries that they become
the primary focus of an extensive, inter-country comparative programme? The first reason is that a large proportion of the rural population of most less developed countries live in communities which show
some or most of the characteristics by which we would define a village:
in India, more than 80 per cent of the population live in villages (Dube,
1958, p. 7). Secondly, villages are usually the primary unit of rural
social organisation: 'the village is a territorial unit, the smallest but
most significant among territorial groups in the social organisation of
the village communities' (Dube, 1955, p. 53). Thirdly, in comparison
with regional studies and studies of kin and caste groups, the village is
a 'relevant manageable unit of analysis' (Berreman, 1972, p. 259).
Villages are easier to delimit than dispersed households, farmsteads or
settlements and form 'useful enumeration groupings' (O'Loughlin,
1972, p. 24) for study of rural households which are often conveniently
located together.

The tentative approaches to a definition of a village have been
neither exhaustive nor exclusive and although the essence of a village is
clear and most studies may be quickly considered relevant or irrelevant,
the definitional fringes are hazy and all cases of doubt have been
included. Sometimes it is often easier to say what a village is not, than
what it is. The term village will more often be applicable to an Indian
community than communities from other countries. For our purposes
– the comparison of behaviour and responses among types of village –
a village is a small, settled group of persons living in and forming almost
all the population of a locality. The actual population of 'a village' is
largely arbitrary as villages vary in size from 50 to 8,000 or more
persons. Most economic, social, political and religious relationships
are formed within the village which can be treated as a behavioural unit.
For nutritional purposes, access to resources (i.e. food) is structured
largely by village prosperity, the distribution of resources and class
relations. The types of food available to each villager will be similar:
villagers usually grow the same crops and purchase the same foods from
the same shops and markets. Thus members of the same village are
likely to eat the same types of food (with the exception of caste
dietary restrictions). Quantities consumed will vary by socio-economic
class and income. Villagers are therefore likely to suffer from the same
type of nutritional deficiency although not to the same extent: cassava

based diets are likely to be protein deficient while maize diets are likely to be deficient in niacin. Finer distinctions such as thiamine deficiencies in all villages which purchase white rice from local mills may be identifiable. Villagers will suffer malnutrition at the same time in villages with no storage facilities, in one-crop villages or in cash-crop villages seasonally cut off from markets (by flooding and lack of transport). For each village these deficiencies may be of the same type (protein-calorie malnutrition in the pre-harvest season or Vitamin A deficiency through lack of green leafy vegetables in the dry season) but degrees of deficiency will differ between villages in response to different socio-economic conditions.

Village membership is by virtue of birth or marriage and the majority of villagers, through having grown up together, have a common background and some common experiences. Most villagers are inevitably members of one or several village institutions such as caste, class or kinship groups and in small villages every villager will know most other village members. The network of social relations is very complex and integrated into a common cultural and social system which at first may seem simple, but in fact forms a series of multiplex relationships that are not specialised to deal with a single activity (F. G. Bailey, 1969, p. 4). A tenant can also be a voter for, debtor to, and tenant, patient and religious follower of his one-man landlord/ politician/moneylender/medical practitioner/religious functionary. Reasons for this multiplicity are inherent in the structure and location of villages: populations are small and therefore contacts are limited; transport is expensive and often non-existent; communications are difficult and public services (education, medical, credit, etc.) are in short supply. Thus, persons of different kinship groups, lineages, castes and sub-castes who are usually set apart are brought together through multiplex relationships, village networks, ties of friendship and loose convivial groupings. Villagers inherit the same culture and physical closeness breeds familiarity with other villagers' food practices. Cooking methods, menus, food preferences and food taboos are common to each village and to villages within definable culture areas.

For both community development and VSP nutritional purposes the functioning of the village as a community is one of its essential attributes. It forms a community by virtue of membership through land tenure, property rights, kinship, etc., but acts as a community through identification, solidarity, common values and interests, communal activities and a multiplicity of relationships. The unity of the village is hidden beneath the separate activities of each caste and each dwelling group and is sometimes temporarily rent by quarrels between individuals or between kin groups. Periodically, however, some event, ceremonial or haphazard, occurs at which the unity of the village is affirmed (Gough, 1955) such as the presence of outsiders and intrusion by Government agents which has important implications for development efforts (Dube 1955). A sense of unity is inevitable since communal use of village wells and trails and communal ownership of grazing land or uncultivated lands promotes solidarity. Villagers have common economic interests: they follow the same agricultural calendar and adverse conditions affect most villagers in the same way. Communal activity is observed in village ceremonies and rituals and in the worship of village gods.

There are of course several problems inherent in the VSP approach including problems of data comparability and reliability. More important is the fact that the village is not always the relevant behavioural unit and that it 'does away with' the effect of the external environment on the lives and decision making processes of the villagers. Many villages cannot be regarded as autonomous, isolated and independent. The idea of economic independence is a myth generated from the study of Indian villages where the economy is founded on the ideal of functional specialisation and interdependence of caste groups. In fact, this economic self-sufficiency is never complete because no village has all the functional occupational groups necessary to maintain its economic existence. Villages are dependent on the external economy while political intervention from outside is frequent. Inter-village caste ties are very important and typical of Indian rural society. They cut across the narrow boundaries of the village and extend over a wide geographical area so that villages are connected through a wide network of social ties of caste membership, marital relations and membership of tribal, religious and other groupings. The village is progressively becoming a part of a wider economy because 'economic relations cut across the boundary of the village in a variety of ways. Many landowners live outside the village. Agricultural surpluses are sold outside. Land has come into the market. Several villagers are engaged in white-collar jobs in the neighbouring towns' (Béteille, 1965, p. 2).

The VSP approach by no means assumes that villages are completely independent. We measure the degree of independence by variables such as land ownership and marketed surplus. However, it became impossible to consider all constraints because the village studies rarely include detailed data on relations between the village and the external environment. The limitations of the VSP are recognised but in attempting to simplify and standardise our framework these limitations have, to some extent, been ignored. The justification lies in the fact that the village is in most cases more an independent than a dependent unit for all the reasons presented earlier in this chapter and because it is the smallest primary unit to which resources are allocated. Villages are far more independent units than farms and anyway the number of village surveys exceeds the number of farm or other micro-level community studies.

A primary aim of the Programme was to collect all the intensive socio-economic surveys of single villages from less developed countries made since 1950, or at least all those that were of some depth, value and reliability. Efforts at retrievement were made by visiting many of the centres producing studies such as Universities, research institutes and government offices in less developed countries and through postal requests. In order to improve on the surveys and provide descriptions of methodology, team members visited authors and fieldworkers in these institutions. These are listed elsewhere (Moore, 1972). Many studies were unpublished and irretrievable as data had not been analysed, tabulated or written up in any usable form. The types and limitations of the village data are discussed in chapter 3; ideally, the most comprehensive village studies provide both data on the village as a functional unit in terms of village facilities, social and kinship structures, etc., and on the characteristics of the village population in terms of land tenure, occupations, etc. Thus a village study providing data for pre-school children only is less comprehensive than a survey providing data on all socio-economic groups by age and sex. These, however, are sometimes included in our research as the availability of village nutrition surveys would otherwise have been greatly reduced. Area studies where the data from several villages are aggregated and farm/settlement surveys of scattered homesteads where the characteristics of the locality or the attributes of the community are not apparent are more easily excluded.

We now have the most comprehensive collection of such village studies available; most are printed and published, but many are available in typescript, photocopy or microfilm form. The existing studies have been carried out for a variety of purposes by researchers of different disciplines working within different organisational structures. Our programme was concerned both with examining and evaluating the methodologies used in obtaining survey data and with producing an operational guide to the methodology of village surveys (see chapter 4). Three papers on the methodology of village studies in less developed countries have been completed (Lipton and Moore, 1972; Schofield, 1972 and Connell, 1973). These evaluate existing survey methods and procedures and detail those methods which appear to obtain the best data while making the most efficient use of available resources.

The next stage of the programme was the preparation of the indexed bibliography which includes a coded entry for each village survey and enables the reader to see at a glance which studies contain data about labour inputs, education, land tenure, nutrition, migration, etc. (Lambert, 1976 and 1978). This indexing was followed by attempts to classify villages by socio-economic variables to form village typologies. Data from about 2,500 studies are being compared to test hypotheses in several related fields of nutrition, demography, education, labour utilisation and migration.

A secondary aim of the project was to find those types of village most likely to respond well to various efforts at improvement and one limited goal was that, for some kinds of input, we should be able to find the sorts of village in which an outlay of given structure and cost would achieve the most of some predefined physical benefit. However, the inherent difficulties in this line of approach soon became apparent and the primary emphasis was limited to the production of village typologies.

The original aims of the nutrition project were as follows: first, to compare food intakes and requirements in different types of village; second, to derive for each village type figures and data on intravillage distribution and to estimate welfare, health and labour quality between villages — differences likely to be related to such physical village characteristics as cropping patterns and such economic characteristics as distribution of land holding; third, to examine the record of nutrition education at village level; and fourth, to use evidence from the analyses to estimate the types of village likely to respond 'best' to alternative measures to improve nutrition. These aims have since been modified due to the paucity of the data.

Conclusions

Planning for better nutrition has, up till now, been a rather haphazard process. It 'does not simply follow a series of textbook steps, but is rather an iterative process that resembles more the tango — four steps forward, three steps back, with an occasional turnaround' (Berg, 1973b, p. 234). New approaches call for procedures which systematically identify and select relevant policy instruments, intervention programmes and nutrition programmes in relation to the causes of malnutrition in the poorly nourished groups.

Until groups with different types of nutrition problem caused by different sets of socio-economic conditions are identified, specific action programmes cannot be implemented and only wasteful 'blanket' programmes can be introduced. There are two problems here: firstly how to identify groups of people and secondly how to define them, by what characteristics and by which variables? Functional and ecological classifications are ways of dividing any country's population into nutritionally vulnerable and 'workable' groups but these do not always fall within well defined units. Villages, on the other hand, are often administrative units in which nutrition programmes can be easily and usefully implemented. The VSP therefore took the village as the primary classification and the VSP approach to the identification of villages by type of diet has been described. In the next chapter we examine the availability and type of micro-level data.

3 AVAILABILITY OF MICRO-LEVEL DATA BY TYPE

Planners have to allocate scarce resources through decisions based on reliable data. Therefore planners often allocate resources to measurement projects and data collection surveys in order to provide data for their substantive decision making. However, they too often ignore or fail to use data which are already available in the form of micro-level village surveys. Planners should retrieve, evaluate and use these second-hand data before filling in gaps by conducting re-surveys or new baseline surveys. Although most micro studies are conducted *ad hoc*, without reference to a general framework of problem identification at the local level, this data search may at best provide an outline for the pattern of nutritional problems within a country. Since 'for many planning situations, a partial answer today is worth a great deal more than a complete answer three years from now' (Berg, 1973b, p. 236), these village data could produce some useful guidelines for identification of (a) types of problems, (b) possible solutions and (c) further research needs.

Therefore we think it essential, before we progress to classifications of village diets, to analyse the types and amounts of available village data. This analysis will show planners what types and how much second-hand material is available and will show the readers what data the results of our research are based upon. In this chapter we discuss the availability of data, the aims of village surveys that have been conducted and the types of data collected. As well as indicating what is already available, such an evaluation will also show the types of data that should be collected in future surveys to enable Governments rationally to allocate their scarce resources for both data collection and programme implementation.

Availability of Village Data

The types of micro-level studies which we in the VSP have been collecting are specific surveys of nutrition in single villages. Approximately 70 per cent of all nutrition-oriented village surveys are available in published form and although we feel confident of having obtained at least 95 per cent of all published articles, we are less certain that most unpublished works have been tapped. Retrieving data by personal visits can be expensive and time consuming. Even so, several field trips to India, Latin America, East and West Africa were undertaken by members of the VSP team. This travel was generously funded by the

25

Table 3.1: Number of Nutrition-Oriented Village Surveys by Area

Area	Number of Village Surveys	Number of Surveyed Villages	Number of Villages per Survey
India	109	201	1.8
Africa	92	247	2.7
Latin America	78	145	1.9
Rest of Asia	39	115	2.9
Oceania	23	52	2.3
Middle East	21	138	6.6
Total	362	898	2.5

Source: Village surveys conducted and published between 1950 and 1973.

Social Science Research Council, the Freedom From Hunger Campaign Committee and the International Labour Organisation. Visits were made to all relevant institutions and a vast amount of unpublished data were collected.

The response rate to written requests for unpublished data varied: enquiries may have been addressed to the wrong people or handled by junior clerks who sent off general information to pacify the retriever; the purpose of the retrieval may have been misunderstood or the material was still in the form of field notes and therefore unavailable. Of all areas in the less developed world, people and institutions in South East Asia were generally very co-operative.

We have retrieved and collected approximately 360 *nutrition-oriented* survey reports which provide data for 900 villages in the less developed world from the Middle East and North Africa, South East Asia, and the Far East, Africa and Latin America[1] (see table 3.1). We have further identified another 82 *general* village surveys which are not specifically nutrition oriented but sometimes provide data on nutritional status. These include 34 surveys from India, 27 from Africa, 3 from Latin America, 16 from Asia (excluding India), 1 from Oceania and 1 from the Middle East. These surveys provide data for another 220 villages.

There are more nutrition specific village surveys available for India than any other area. These represent 30 per cent of the total surveys; 25 per cent were conducted in Africa; 22 per cent in Latin America; 11 per cent in Asia (excluding India); 6 per cent in Oceania and 6 per cent in the Middle East. However, more villages have been surveyed in Africa than any other area and the village to survey ratio is 2.7 : 1. This ratio is highest for the Middle East (6.6 : 1) since the regional surveys incorporate numerous villages for which the data are disaggregated. The mean village to survey ratio is 2.5 villages per survey.

However, these figures are distorted because not all surveys provide data which are either reliable or useful. For VSP purposes, the number of Indian villages with useful nutrition data was limited to 47 because the household samples were often unrepresentative of the village. Three types of Indian survey can be identified: firstly, socio-economic studies by the Agro-Economic Research Centres (AERCs) and the Census of India Surveys. These are non-nutrition oriented research institutes and the surveys provide mainly qualitative, descriptive nutrition data and some other data on subjects relevant to nutrition such as crop production and marketing. Secondly, surveys with the primary objective of collecting health data. These have been conducted by the Planning Research and Action Institute, Lucknow, Uttar Pradesh; the Narangwal Rural Health Research Centre, Punjab, and the Rural Health Training Centre, Sarojini Nagar. Thirdly, nutrition surveys conducted by teams of individuals from nutrition research institutes, Universities and Home Science colleges whose location has heavily biased the sample of village specific nutrition surveys in favour of certain states including Madras, Andhra Pradesh and Gujarat. The main institutes we contacted were the National Institute of Nutrition, Hyderabad, Andhra Pradesh; the Sri Avinashilingham Home Science College, Coimbatore, Madras; the Christian Science Medical College, Vellore, Madras, and the Lady Irwin Home Science College, Delhi, Gujarat.

The village studies conducted under the auspices of these Institutes usually follow a uniform pattern. Many of the surveys from the National Institute of Nutrition are 'experimental' and hypothesis testing, providing specific data for the formulation of nutrition programmes. These studies are rarely intensive socio-economic surveys of a single village although the subjects are often villagers from the Telegana region of Andhra Pradesh. Theses from the Coimbatore Home Science College are fairly uniform but concentrate on vulnerable groups. They often provide useful food and nutrient consumption data for individual families but the samples are usually small and the socio-economic conditions of each family are not described in detail. The implementation and evaluation of standardised Nutrition Education programmes is a primary objective of most of these studies although the villages in which these programmes are implemented are fairly close to the college and the frequency and closeness of contacts may well bias the survey results. Data from these theses often provide material for the articles published from this Institute. Other village nutrition surveys are conducted in each state by the Directorate General of Health Services. These are usually only available in mimeograph form and are difficult to obtain.

The VSP has systematically searched all the AERC material and all

available volumes of the 1961 Census of India. The majority of the
Census reports provide only qualitative data but this information,
together with data on vital statistics, availability and use of medical
facilities, environmental sanitation, child-rearing practices, etc.
complements other village surveys providing mainly nutrition data.
The Census surveys often provide crop production, consumption and
sales data usable in food balance sheet exercises. The results may not
be altogether accurate, but are sometimes useful as Nair (1961) and
Yeshwanth (1964) show in their similar treatment of the University of
Madras AERC material. Some of these AERC studies provide very
useful expenditure data, sometimes broken down into cereal and
non-cereal foods. Data on personal hygiene, sanitation and types of
food consumed are also included.

The majority of village studies for the rest of Asia are mainly
health oriented. They concentrate on assessing the incidence of diseases
and infestations or on measuring nutritional status (often of specific
groups) through anthropometry. Food consumption and other
nutrition data are sometimes included but are often descriptive and of
poor quality. Village-specific nutrition surveys are few in number and
those by Hauck and Bailey (for a synopsis, see Bailey, 1964 and Hauck,
1959) are the exceptions. These are notable for the provision of
reliable and extensive food/nutrient consumption data.

The Asian surveys are distributed between four main areas: Indonesia, Thailand, Philippines and Malaysia. For other countries
(Bangladesh, Nepal, Pakistan, Sri Lanka, etc.) very few surveys have
been located and/or retrieved. The predominance of data from Thailand
is due to the large number of reports provided by the South East Asia
Programme at Cornell University. Some of these studies represent the
best nutrition-specific village studies available. Collectively they provide
a vast amount of data for one village. The University of the Philippines,
the Community Development Research Council, the World Health
Organisation's Regional Office for the Western Pacific and the Institute
for Medical Research in Malaysia are important sources of village data
in Asia. Surveys conducted by the Food and Nutrition Research Center,
Manila, though of outstanding quality, were discarded as non-village
specific.

Unlike many of the Asian studies (with the exception of India)
surveys from Oceania are nutrition oriented and tend to include health
and anthropometric data. Most of the surveys are fairly old (1950s)
baseline surveys which provide data rather than test hypotheses. The
two main areas of study are the Cook Islands and Papua New Guinea
where community studies predominate but do not qualify as village
surveys. However, one of the few surveys available on energy intake and
expenditure is from this area and deserves special mention as a useful

and original piece of research (Hipsley and Kirk, 1965). Large amounts of unpublished data from Oceania are unavailable even in mimeo form because staff and resources for calculation, tabulation and presentation are inadequate. The New Guinea Research Institute is a particularly useful data source. The South Pacific Commission and South Pacific Health Service provide data for other areas in Oceania.

In general, the African studies are of a better quality than those from other areas. They provide more village data and often assess nutritional status by clinical, biochemical and anthropometric parameters as well as through diet surveys. Unlike the Indian village studies which concentrate on vulnerable groups, the African surveys disaggregate data by age groups, while surveys devoted to the study of the nutritional status of pregnant and lactating women are rare. Surveys of the pre-school village population are more common. In comparison with India, fewer theses have been retrieved, but these are of a better quality and a few of them are particularly outstanding. The ORSTOM (Office de la Récherche Scientifique et Technique Outre Mer) studies are especially detailed and have been retrieved for the Cameroons, Togo, the Congo and the Ivory Coast. Most of these French studies provide useful data on seasonal consumption patterns.

A large number of the African studies were conducted in Nigeria, Tanzania and Gambia. In Nigeria, good data are provided by the Food Science and Applied Nutrition Unit at the University of Ibadan and in studies conducted by Morley (1968), Nicol (1956 and 1959) and Collis (1962); in the Gambia a vast amount of data are available for Keneba village; in Tanzania health surveys seem to predominate. The Cameroons, Senegal, Ghana and Uganda provide the next most important set of studies.

Some of the useful institutes in Africa include the Department of Community Health, Nairobi; the University of Ibadan, Nigeria; the East African Institute for Medical Research, Tanzania; Makerere Medical School, Kampala; the FAO Regional Office for Africa, Accra; Organisme de Récherche sur l'Alimentation et la Nutrition Africaines (ORANA), Dakar and the various ORSTOM centres.

Relatively few Latin American village studies have been retrieved by the Village Studies Project because Latin American community studies are not, by our definition, village studies. However, we have collected those which most closely resemble village surveys. The quality and quantity of Guatemalan surveys exceeds those from other Latin American countries primarily because INCAP (Institute de Nutrición de Centro América y Panamá) headquarters are located there. Scrimshaw, Flores and others (1957–65) have conducted intensive, longitudinal studies in three towns selected by INCAP which are extremely good. Other useful surveys are available for Jamaica, Peru and Puerto Rico. For countries like Chile, Costa Rica, French Guiana, Guyana, Honduras, Nicaragua and Surinam, very few, if any, surveys have been conducted. We found that Brazilian studies are predominantly health oriented, those from Peru are numerous, nutrition oriented and include some of the few child-care studies available; studies in Puerto Rico provide useful data on the intra-household distribution of foods and nutrients and the best Jamaican studies investigate the relationship between child growth and factors in the social environment. The National Institutes of Nutrition are often the only useful sources of nutrition data in some countries including Bolivia, Columbia, Ecuador and Mexico. Survey methods are common and data are presented in a standardised format.

In comparison with Africa, Latin America and India, relatively few village surveys have been collected from the Middle East. Most available surveys from this area were conducted in the United Arab Republic and Iran. In the UAR, most of the retrieved surveys are health oriented and concerned with determining the incidence of helminthic and protozoal infections such as diarrhoea. However, our information is somewhat biased by the non-retrieval of a series of surveys conducted by the Institute of Nutrition, Cairo. For Iran, there is a predominance of nutrition surveys organised jointly by the FAO and the Food and Nutrition Institute of Teheran. These attempt to assess the food consumption and nutrition situation of one area instead of individual villages but in doing so usually provide data for about 10 or more villages. Socio-economic data are not usually provided for each village and recommendations are made for areas rather than villages. One of the best Iranian surveys was conducted under the auspices of the Gorg-Tapeh Centre for Rural Nutrition, Education and Research and this provided quite detailed data for several villages and especially for Gorg-Tapeh (Hedayat, 1969). Few surveys are available for Lebanon and Turkey.

Survey Aims

It is useful to identify two types of aim: the primary objective which specifies the main area of data collection and the secondary aim which specifies the intended use of the data after collection. If the intended uses of the study are clear (to eliminate worms and thus improve nutrition) so are the study objectives (to assess worm infestation and the costs of curing it). Often, however, intended use is either lacking or inappropriate. Lack of secondary aims indicates that little thought has been given to the use of the data and that a large bank of information is available which may or may not be used by planners. If it is not used, then the time and money spent on data collection is wasted.

Unfortunately, we had to infer (or guess) the goals of most of the surveys from the data collected which in itself suggests that survey aims

Table 3.2: Percentage of Different Types of Village Survey by Area

Area	Total no. of Surveys	Nutritional Status %	Food Consumption %	Physical Status %
India	109	47.7	44	8.3
Africa	92	50	23.9	26.1
Latin America	78	46.2	23.1	30.8
Rest of Asia	39	30.8	35.9	33.3
Oceania	23	65.2	17.4	17.4
Middle East	21	61.9	4.8	33.3
Total	362	48.1	29.6	22.4

need to be more clearly elucidated. We found that surveys which were not providing baseline data for a nutrition programme or were not eventually to give rise to a resurvey generally lacked secondary aims, at least in the short run, whereas the policy purposes of resurveys were usually clearer. One-off surveys were likely to be most useful if they aimed to test some particular hypothesis.

Types of Survey

Three types were identified: firstly, 'food consumption' surveys which provide data on food and nutrient intakes; secondly, 'nutritional status' surveys which provide both food consumption data and anthropometric, clinical or biochemical data; and thirdly, 'physical status' surveys which provide only anthropometric, clinical or biochemical data. The percentages of each type of survey by area are included in table 3.2.

We can also classify surveys as baseline surveys or resurveys. Baseline surveys either provide general data on the nutritional situation of the village, are specific surveys which assess the incidence of the type of nutritional deficiency, or provide programme specific data for the introduction of some type of intervention. The purpose of resurveys is usually clearer. They may be the natural follow-up to earlier baseline surveys being designed to evaluate change in nutritional status, food consumption and health over a period of time, even if no programme has been introduced, or they may be introduced as evaluatory surveys to assess the impact of a nutritional improvement programme.

Baseline surveys are more common than resurveys for several reasons: firstly, there is a long time lag between the publication of the baseline and resurvey results; secondly, resurvey data are often not published; thirdly, the number of resurveys is too small for any reliable conclusions to be drawn and there is no incentive to produce 'just one more'; fourthly, improvement programmes are implemented in villages

Table 3.3: Percentage of Baseline Surveys and Resurveys by Area

Area	Total Number of Surveys	Percentage of Baseline Surveys	Percentage of Resurveys
India	109	63.3	36.7
Africa	92	94.6	5.4
Latin America	78	84.6	15.4
Rest of Asia	39	89.7	10.3
Oceania	23	95.7	4.3
Middle East	21	90.5	9.5

other than those initially surveyed and their impact evaluated through aggregate changes in nutritional status. Village resurveys are popular in India and are very infrequently conducted in Oceania and Africa. This is because many of the Indian surveys are experimental, hypothesis testing and evaluative. The impact of applied nutrition programmes, feeding programmes and vitamin supplementation programmes are evaluated at the village level more frequently in India than elsewhere. In Africa the impact of nutrition intervention programmes is often evaluated at the regional rather than the village level.

As a guideline to the probability of using baseline data in the future, the baseline:resurvey ratio can be calculated. This was found to be very high for Oceania (22:1) and Africa (17.4:1) and less for Latin America (5.5:1), Asia (8.8:1) and the Middle East (9.5:1). The ratio was lowest for India (1.7:1) where nearly 50 per cent of the resurveys were conducted by MSc students as part of their dissertation. These were often brief and conducted after the implementation of short Nutrition Education programmes.

At any given time the number of baseline surveys exceeds the number of resurveys. For recent baseline surveys not enough time will have elapsed to allow for programme completion and the conducting of resurveys. However, many of the baseline surveys published between 1950 and 1970 were carried out before 1965 which leaves a space of six years for programme implementation and evaluation. This is not unrealistic in view of some of the resurveys which have been completed. Fifty per cent of the baseline surveys were conducted between 1960 and 1965, while 49 per cent of the resurveys were conducted between 1965 to 1969. This implies a gap of approximately five years between the initial baseline survey and the resurvey. Analysis of the Indian data on its own reveals a similar time lag of three to five years. If this is the standard time lag we should expect few new resurveys to appear because comparatively few baseline surveys were conducted between 1967 and 1970.

Types of Survey Data

Data collected in village surveys includes *indirect* data which are vital
statistics indicating problem villages or areas but not their cause (malnutrition, infection or both) and *proximate* data which provide us with
evidence on the direct physical reasons for poor nutritional status
(unbalanced or insufficient diet). *Ultimate* data suggests causes, other
than proximate ones (lack of food) for the presence or absence of
problems, by size and type. Thus high infant mortality rates are
indirect data which will lead planners to suspect a nutrition and health
problem. Proximate data for the same village may then provide
evidence of an underweight population with a large calorie deficit and
marasmic children. But the real causes of the calorie deficit (we know
it must be caused by lack, waste or maldistribution of calorie foods)
remain unknown until further ultimate data are made available on
cropping patterns, man/land ratios, presence or absence of retail inlets,
income levels, etc., i.e. 'the factors which underlie and influence food
consumption' (Reh, 1962).

Indirect Data

Infant mortality rates, if reliable, are a useful and cheap indicator of
health status. They are a pointer to areas of nutritional and health
problems, but only indicate the area of problem location and do not
measure its size or type. These data are available in Census Statistics
and other regional or national sample surveys. Unfortunately they are
not always reliable as data on some deaths, particularly in the neonatal
period, are especially difficult to obtain. General village surveys can
provide more reliable data of this type but nutrition surveys are usually
conducted so quickly that there is not enough time to collect these
data. Infant mortality rates are available for 31, 9, 5, 11, 22 and 4 per
cent of the villages from the Middle East, Oceania, South East Asia,
India, Africa and Latin America respectively.

Proximate Data

Type and reliability of proximate data varies between surveys. Many
studies would benefit from the services of a statistician since samples
are frequently too small and some surveys, notably the Indian ones,
only provide proximate data for traditionally vulnerable sections of the
population. These data are not therefore always representative of the
village.

　　Food consumption data are generally incomplete which inhibits any
type of comparative analysis of survey results. Absence of data on
alcohol consumption is especially striking since this is often an important source of calories and D vitamins which may be available to only
a small section of the population (adults). Food staples used in the

preparation of these beverages are thus diverted away from other members of the family/village. Data are most frequently available on the types of staples consumed but data on fruit, vegetable and legume consumption are not always given. These are sometimes aggregated by food groups which is not very useful if the reader wants to calculate the percentage of nutrients provided by each category of food. Data on food sources are equally poor. Ideally, surveys should provide two sets of results: one for home produced and one for purchased food. Seasonal data are rare and even descriptive data on seasonal variations are absent.

Qualitative data are often omitted or include descriptions of food habits, taboos, meal patterns, cooking practices, menus, etc., which are usually superficial and brief. This is unfortunate since the data are easy to collect and could provide useful information to either reinterpret quantitative results or to contribute to the bulk of qualitative food knowledge. Surveys should present these data even when they do not directly bear on the primary and secondary aims of the survey because reader requirements are varied or unknown. Data on food wastage, for example, are rarely included but could indicate the potential value of the diet.

Most of the food and nutrient consumption data are given in mean figures per head, per day or in terms of consumption coefficients which do not take into account the intra-family maldistribution of foods. Nutrient requirements are rarely calculated and diet adequacies usually assessed by comparison with standardised recommended allowances. But this is dangerous as international standards are only an approximation and have to be handled carefully: Nicol (1956) found that the weights and heights of Ibo and Yoruba children were less than the American and British standards, although their diets supplied about 18 per cent more calories and protein than the allowances recommended by the FAO. It was inferred that the allowances were not sufficient for these children's needs, owing to the additional requirements caused by environmental factors of temperature and humidity, infestation with intestinal parasites and malaria. Thus 'field measurement of food requirements in relation to physical activity and environmental stresses along with studies of the associated biochemical and functional changes are needed' (Oluwasanmi, 1966, p. 69). Nutritionists should prepare and use local standards for different ethnic groups and 'it is particularly desirable to collect reliable present-day local standards for young children' (Jelliffe, 1966, p. 54). National tables for nutrient requirements are frequently used but should still be adjusted for local conditions. At very least, rough correction factors — to allow for type of local work, climate, population structure, etc. — should be used with international and national tables.

Nutrient requirements vary between villages by up to 400 calories (Nicol, 1959). To emphasise this, we have calculated the calorie requirements for two hypothetical villages. The difference was found to be as great as 2,147 calories per head per day (see Appendix B). However, village requirements, if calculated, are rarely presented and cannot be recalculated because proximate data on physiological status (including data on sex, age, weight and height), pathogenic status, the climate and labour inputs are usually absent. The energy expended on physical activities accounts for a high proportion of the total requirement for calories but requirement calculations do not accurately account for variations with the type and intensity of labour inputs since very little is known about the energy cost of different activities. At best, adult males and females are classified as sedentary, moderate or active but these categories assume a consistent level of energy expenditure throughout the year. The recommended allowances also assume that adolescent and even younger family members do not expend at least some calories on agricultural or other work.

Ramanamurthy (1966) calculated the metabolic cost of eight agricultural activities for Indian labourers of which trimming bunds cost 9.3 calories per kg body weight per hour, making irrigation channels 4.56 cals/kg per hour and ploughing 7.02 cals/kg per hour. Cleave (1970) found that in Africa, cultivation (which includes ploughing and hoeing) requires 4.9 cals/kg body weight per hour, weeding requires 3.4 and picking 2.0 calories/kg body weight per hour while Fox (1953) found that in Gambia, the calorie cost of farm activities varied between 95 to 315 calories per hour per man. In West Africa, Phillips (1954) also found a great variation in the calorie costs of different jobs: 269 calories per hour for grass cutting, 274 for hoeing, 360 for sowing, 372 for bush clearing and 504 for tree felling.

Some crops are more labour intensive per cultivated acre than others and variations in energy expenditure between villages and over time are closely defined by the cropping pattern. Thus certain types of village will have higher or seasonal work requirements for calories than other types of village. A mono-crop, single cropping village with a seasonal labour peak, and consistent levels of employment and workforce dependent ratios will have different energy requirements from a multi-crop, continuous cropping village with a highly migrant workforce population. Dispersal of land holdings will also make a difference as Fox (1953) found in Gambia where 23.3 per cent of the energy expended for millet cultivation was spent on walking to and from the fields compared with 4.4 per cent for groundnuts and 14 per cent for rice. The cost of energy expenditure is especially important if seasonal demands for labour coincide with seasonal food shortages. This situation can result in loss of body weight, reduced work output, lower yields and therefore even worse food shortages in the next agricultural year as Fox found in Gambia where the 'intensity of effort required in their work exhausted their available energy, causing an early onset of fatigue and thus limiting the total time they were able to work' (1953, p. 76). However, data on the size of labour inputs are sparse in village nutrition studies (only 10 per cent of the African and one per cent of the surveys from Oceania provide those data).

Ultimate Data

Far worse than gaps in proximate data is the lack of 'ultimate' data about the socio-economic causes of inadequate nutrition without which relevant solutions cannot be found. Unless these causes are identified and dealt with, new resource inputs − of any type − will be as prone to their effects as are food resources already in the village. More food may be made available by new inputs, but increasing total availability is no use if the disadvantaged sections of the village population fail to benefit as a result of unchanged causal factors like maldistribution (between or within families or over time) or culturally determined food habits. Problems of intra-household distribution will still be incurred and if cooking habits prevent the parboiling of rice, food beliefs channel low protein foods towards ill people and food taboos affect the nutritionally most vulnerable groups, any attempts at fortification or supplementation may be destroyed. Whether it is the lack of ultimate data which has restricted the types of improvement programmes, or whether the latter were never designed to tackle the ultimate factors is another problem. The fact that nutrition education programmes have attempted to change some social and cultural variables affecting food consumption shows that some importance is attached to the ultimate causes of poor nutrition. However, without clearly identifying those ultimate factors, these programmes are often ineffective: many nutrition education programmes do not know what to teach and are perhaps never aimed at the most important target groups.

Agro-economic, environmental and social factors affect both the need for nutrients and levels of food intake. Until these are identified (see table 3.4) long-term solutions cannot be chosen with any degree of reliability. Village food availability is affected by these factors, the most important being on-farm production of food for family consumption (which we term 'subsistence productivity', using the words in a rather specific sense), purchasing power of non-subsistence output and resource distribution in the village.

Subsistence productivity depends mainly on the area and quality of village lands, their ownership, agricultural techniques, the size of the

Table 3.4: Percentage of Villages from Each Area with Data on Factors Affecting Subsistence Food Production

	Africa	India	Rest of South-East Asia (excluding India)	Latin America	Middle East	Oceania
Land area	0	5	0	2	16	1
Land use (cropping patterns, crop calendar and rotation)	6	3	6	0	3	0
Land tenure (distribution of owned and operated land, tenure and rent arrangements, fragmentation of holdings)	3	4	2	0	6	0
Rainfall	16	14	7	8	6	8
Altitude	17	6	15	28	12	8
Terrain	30	13	23	22	12	13
Soil	17	7	12	8	22	8
Occupational patterns	18	78	53	10	15	17
Agricultural labour inputs and labour productivity	8	0	0	0	0	1
Use of fertilisers, manure, new seeds, extension	1	46	0	1	0	0
Presence or absence of different types of co-operatives and credit institutions[a]	1	2	0	1	3	0
Membership and use of co-operatives	1	0	0	0	0	0
Agricultural techniques (mechanisation, use of animal traction, composting, threshing, etc.)	6	1	0	0	3	0
Means and extent of irrigation	5	10	1	1	3	0
Main agricultural produce	23	14	23	17	16	2
Subsistence produce[b]	14	14	31	3	6	23
Cash produce[c]	20	3	16	9	3	3
Fodder[d]	0	0	0	0	3	0
Quantity of farm output	6	8	0	1	0	0
Value of farm output	2	0	0	0	0	0
Marketing and storage arrangements[e]	0	13	6	1	0	2
Ownership of livestock	19	9	2	4	0	1

Source: Village surveys conducted and published between 1950 and 1971.

Notes:

[a] The co-operative include marketing co-operatives, service co-operatives and credit co-operatives: they affect the level of agricultural investment and inputs by the provision of credit, seeds, fertilisers, etc., which should increase agricultural production.

[b] Includes surveys where, although subsistence produce as such is not mentioned, one could ascertain this data from food intake data.

[c] The ratio of cash crops to subsistence crops is an important factor in determining food availability and labour requirements, especially in Africa, where the harvesting of cash crops occurs at times of food scarcity.

[d] Fodder crops may not be grown in the village, as cattle may not be kept. The lack of fodder crops in villages which keep cattle may affect food supplies.

[e] This includes data on the quantities marketed, marketing prices, types of marketing arrangements, time of marketing and length of storage and mode of crop storage.

labour force and the use of working time which is governed by employment patterns and job conditions within and outside the village. The amount and type of inputs along with other ecological factors, like climate and soil types, affect productivity. These factors will determine the types of subsistence crop, the size of the output and cropping patterns (the number of crops per year and the seasonality of cropping and crop rotations). The timing and number of harvests will, together with output, determine post-harvest food availability. Only if adequate storage facilities exist or continuous, staggered or multiple cropping patterns obviate the need for storage facilities can food be adequately distributed throughout the year (even if enough is produced to feed the village until the next harvest). In spite of the importance of these data, information in village surveys is poor (table 3.4). More data are provided on the type of village produce and local conditions than on land use/area/tenure, labour inputs or farm output because they are easier to collect.

If subsistence productivity is inadequate or lacking in variety, food has to be purchased. Levels of purchase are governed by (a) cash incomes, in relation to (b) food prices, (c) food expenditure patterns and (d) the prices of, and preferences of villagers among non-food purchases. Cash income is affected by the extent to which village products are sold, the market value of non-subsistence output, the job opportunities within and outside the village, migration patterns, and the extent to which labour can be freed from agricultural employment in the village in order to find alternative job opportunities. The village studies show that the rural combination of farming for subsistence with subsidiary employment has considerable attraction in that it avoids the temptation of farming for cash at the expense of subsistence production and it also provides an alternative economic pursuit for the farmers during the slack agricultural period. However, in the lowest income groups, a decline in income may well affect the diet less than fluctuations of income over the year. In either case, cash supplementation of subsistence foodstuffs will not be feasible unless there are facilities (retail inlets and markets) for the purchase of food. Data on factors affecting food purchase are more frequent than data on factors affecting productivity (see tables 3.4 and 3.5) but on their own are still not useful. For example, information on village location tells us nothing until we can establish some reliable and useful relationship between village accessibility, location and purchasing patterns. More data on food sources and the timing and quantity of food purchase would provide a useful guide to factors affecting food sources and indicate trends in purchasing patterns.

It is not enough to examine the availability of food within the village. We must also examine *food distribution* which affects the

Table 3.5: Percentage of Villages from each Area with Data on Factors Affecting Food Availability in the Cash Sphere

	Africa	India	Rest of South East Asia (excluding India)	Latin America	Middle East	Oceania
Distance from nearest town	23	41	17	13	41	5
Communications[a]	16	38	10	23	3	12
Retail inlets	17	5	2	7	16	2
Food sources (produced or purchased)	10	14	6	11	0	5
Incomes	10	43	5	9	6	0
Food expenditure patterns	10	21	5	9	0	0
Food prices	5	2	0	4	0	0

Source: Village surveys conducted and published between 1950 and 1971.
Note:
[a] These include the presence or absence of roads (including the distance from main roads and railway halts) and motorised public transport. Such factors limit the import and export of food; transportation problems are often responsible for high food losses.

adequacy of diet along three dimensions: between villages; among households within a village and within households. Inter-village distribution will be governed by factors affecting food availability such as village isolation, the availability of markets, distance from towns, etc. Inter-household distribution is governed by income levels, land size, household size, etc., while intra-household distribution is affected by family size, the number of children, the number of wives, meal patterns, eating habits and food beliefs (see chapter 6). Data on all these factors are poor. Even though the household is the major unit for data collection, only a small proportion of surveys provide data on household size and/or composition and structure.

Conclusions

Socio-economic and specific nutritional/health studies of single villages are one of the primary sources of micro-level nutrition data in less developed countries and should be referred to by planners in the formulation and implementation of any country's nutrition policy. To facilitate this, we have made a collection of these surveys and produced an annotated bibliography of village nutrition studies which is now available for planners and/or research workers to use.

Ideally, surveys should provide all or most of the data needed to allow users to both evaluate the reliability of the results and re-use the data for purposes different from those of the survey. Unfortunately, crucial and easily obtainable data such as sample size are often omitted so that it is difficult to re-use the data. Publishing space is an obvious constraint on the amount of data that can be included, but published articles should at least specify, for interested users, where the original data are available. If there are no constraints on the amount of material that can be included in the unpublished report, then authors should be less restrictive on what they include. The situation is even more serious if resources are so scarce that data are not thoroughly analysed or written up in a form usable by other people unfamiliar with the data. Here, international organisations could help by providing teams and facilities for data analysis. Overworked project organisers and harassed field workers could send data to a central organisation which could analyse the data and keep a set of results for a central data bank.

Methods of analysis and sources of data (especially of recommended nutrient allowances) should always be included as this will enable the reader to (a) make comparisons between surveys using different methods of data collection and (b) assess for himself its reliability. Survey evaluation need not always be lengthy and even vague statements like 'the dietary survey may not have been accurate to within 400 to 500 cal.' (Nicol, 1956, p. 194) are better than none at all. Familiarity both with the data and general village conditions should enable the author to suggest reasons for deficiencies and methods for nutritional improvement using village resources whenever possible. Not all village nutrition surveys have to be policy-oriented but the purest of research must suggest, to a competent researcher, some implications for policy which are worth sharing with his readers.

More surveys include data on both food consumption and physical measures of health status than on either consumption or nutritional status alone. The survey aims are often not clearly stated and have to be inferred from the data, making it impossible to assess the methods of data collection within the framework of the study objectives. Ideally, surveys should be conducted on the basis of both primary objectives, in terms of descriptive data gathering and hypothesis testing, and secondary aims, or intended uses of the survey results. Both goals should make the best possible use of research resources in support of policy. The disproportionately greater number of baseline surveys suggests the need for more careful resource allocation and closer links between initial measurements, interventions and evaluative resurveys. The existence of a vast amount of information which looks as if it will not be 'used' also indicates the necessity for closer links between nutrition policy planners and institutions conducting surveys. This will ensure that all survey results are distributed to planners or that surveys are not conducted without the approval of planners or without the applied aims being stated beforehand. Because nutrition surveys are conducted by a variety of people and institutions, without reference to an overall planning frame, it might be most practical to process all nutrition survey results in a central data bank.

Analysis of village survey data showed that most of the data were proximate; indirect data were rarely included and ultimate (causative) data more rarely still. There were gaps in the proximate data especially on the intra-village and intra-household distribution of foods, but lack of ultimate data seriously hinders the development and implementation of types of improvement programme. Choice of programme is limited to (for example), supplementation or fortification, but not irrigation or improved storage, let alone land reform. The allocation of nutritional resources such as skimmed milk powder or fortified bread to villagers will tackle the proximate causes of nutritional deficiencies but will not improve the ultimate, causal factors: if these remain unchanged, the free milk powder may not even reach the vulnerable target groups, while neglect of causal factors may lead to 'cures worse than the disease'. For example, costly fortified bread, if the poor are persuaded to buy it, can use up their cash and leave them with fewer calories than before.

Until more comprehensive socio-economic nutritional village studies have been conducted, it is difficult to suggest types of ultimate data to be collected. It would be a waste of resources to collect each and every type if it could be shown that information on a few key variables would facilitate the implementation of improvement programmes. Since less developed countries do not have the financial resources to collect information on all these variables, we would suggest that firstly, present conductors of intensive socio-economic surveys put more effort into collecting reliable and useful data on nutrition variables. This would provide more nutrition data without putting any extra strain on existing resources. Secondly, instead of surveying numerous villages to a rather superficial level, research institutes conducting socio-economic surveys should allocate more of their available resources to more effective sampling, re-surveying and more detailed analysis of the data in a smaller sample of villages. Thirdly, we suggest that nutritional resources allocated to measurement surveys should be distributed towards in-depth nutritional studies of fewer villages rather than shallow nutritional investigation of more villages. In line with the general VSP approach, we suggest fourthly, that types of data we have discussed should be collected for a few villages with identifiable nutritional problems. Once we have identified the socio-economic causes of nutritional problem by area or type of village, the cost of nutritional assessment is negligible. Thus, we are not suggesting that in poor countries, more resources should be allocated to nutritional measurement and identification of ultimate data. This would be nice, but we also believe that better and more useful data could be obtained within the existing resource structure provided that resources are used more realistically and efficiently. Instead of spending money on expensive food consumption surveys in one area, it may be more efficient to assess the nutritional situation by cheaper methods and spend more time and money collecting information on firstly, domestic systems including family decision making; size and timing of labour inputs of different types from various sources (including females and children); child care by season; family structure, size and type especially in relation to child and infant malnutrition. Secondly, agricultural systems to determine how the use of given farm resources, in space and time, affects food availability; cropping patterns in relation to seasonality; size and type of crop output; walking distance to fields and the type of agricultural economy (subsistence or cash). Thirdly, economic systems to study the influence of cash versus subsistence food production; the balance of workers to dependants; food availability and distribution; migration; intra- and extra-village job opportunities; income levels and the seasonality of employment. Fourthly, environmental systems, to find out whether to remove health constraints or to attempt alternative improvements; sanitation facilities; types and quality of water supply; house types; types of cooking facilities; overcrowding; presence or absence of village health facilities; degree of village isolation in terms of presence of roads, motorised transport, etc. Fifthly, ecological models to identify regions characterised by types of nutrition problem: data on terrain, soil types, climate, ecology, etc.

Note

1. The countries covered in each area include for the Middle East and North Africa: Algeria, Iran, Israel, Lebanon, Sudan, United Arab Republic and the Yemen Arab Republic. In South-East Asia village surveys are available for Bangladesh, Cambodia, India, Indonesia, Laos, Malaysia, Nepal, Pakistan Philippines, Sri Lanka, Thailand and Vietnam. For the Far East surveys are available for the Caroline Islands, Cook Islands, Fiji Islands, Papua New Guinea and Samoa. Africa includes the Cameroons, Central African Republic, Chad, Comores, Congo, Ethiopia, Gambia, Ghana, Guinea, Ivory Coast, Kenya, Mali, Malagas, Malawi, Nigeria, Senegal, Tanzania, Togo, Uganda and the Upper Volta. For Latin America the countries for which village studies are available include Bolivia, Brazil, Chile, Colombia, Dominica, Ecuador, Guatemala, Haiti, Jamaica, Mexico, Nicaragua, Panama, Peru, Puerto Rico, Uruguay and Venezuela.

4 METHODS OF DATA COLLECTION

In order to assess the reliability and comparability of village nutrition surveys an enquiry was mounted into the methods of data collection. Economic surveys, food consumption surveys and medical surveys which provide direct evidence, usually quantitative, of the size and type of nutrition problem were at once identified. Other surveys provide indirect evidence of malnutrition which indicate rather than directly measure problems. These include surveys providing vital statistics and descriptive surveys of food consumption.

Methods Used in Surveys of Different Types

Assessment of a nutritional situation can be achieved through using one or a combination of several methods. Since the literature on these is abundant, we will only provide a brief description of these here. For a lengthier summary see Schofield (1972).

Food Balance Sheets are commonly used by the UN Food and Agricultural Organisation at national and regional levels. At the micro level this method does not provide any reliable indication of the number of people actually suffering from malnutrition and at best only allows rough inter-village comparisons of food availability. Similarly, *Economic Surveys* (patterns and levels of food expenditure) are only indicative of whether families can or cannot afford to purchase an adequate diet. *Food Consumption Surveys* provide data on the types and amounts of foods consumed by a representative sample of the survey population. The nutrient content of the foods is calculated from standard food composition tables and individual, *per capita* or nutrient intakes per consumption unit are calculated and compared with recommended allowances to provide evidence of nutrient gaps. There are several methods used in food consumption surveys: the *Food Weighment Method* involves measuring the amounts of foods (both raw and cooked) consumed at each meal, taking into account food wasted in preparation and left-overs. Individual portions can be painstakingly measured or total family intake is weighed and individual intakes calculated from consumption coefficients. *Food Composite Analysis* is even more precise: aliquot portions of all meals consumed are obtained and their nutrient content chemically determined. A less precise method is *Recall* which relies on the housewife remembering the amounts of foods consumed by the family over a specified time period. The housewife may be required to use standardised measuring units to indicate the size of the raw and cooked ingredients consumed, or the

43

investigator may permit her to indicate these by using household utensils whose capacity must be determined.

Another method based on the same principle as the food balance sheet is the *Inventory* or *Log Book Method*. The fieldworker weighs the amount of food available in the household at the beginning of the survey and leaves the scales with the housewife who records the weights of all foods brought into the household during the survey period. Food left in the household at the end of the survey is weighed by the investigator and the family food consumption over the survey period can then be approximated. Less refined and cruder methods of measuring food consumption exist and include the construction of *Food Lists* in order to determine the type and frequency of food consumption. Similarly *Diet Histories* can be obtained by questionnaire.

The data provided by *Medical Surveys* varies in reliability from precise biochemical and anthropometric information to data on the incidence of deficiency diseases. Depletion of body stores is the first stage in the development of deficiency diseases and some biochemical methods assay the level of nutrients in body fluids. For example serum protein and albumin levels indicate the level of protein malnutrition and other blood analyses include assessments of the serum Vitamin A, Vitamin C and Iron.

Clinical Examinations provide data on the incidence of deficiency symptoms but since the identification of nutrient deficiencies depends upon slight differences in colour and texture, dryness and pigmentation, it is not always easy to attribute one particular symptom to the absence of certain nutrients in the diet. Severe nutritional deficiency disease is easily recognisable and so is robust good health but it is the identification of the marginal cases (perhaps 90 per cent of the total) which is difficult. Deficiency symptoms may be absent even though nutrient deficits exist or symptoms may be the delayed result of previous deficiencies in intake. For example, symptoms observed in post-harvest periods of food availability are more likely to reflect deficiencies suffered in the previous period of food shortage. Thus biochemical tests should be conducted on a subsample of those clinically examined to confirm the extent of the deficiency.

Anthropometric Data is the most important criterion for judging nutritional status in infancy and childhood. The triceps skinfold, weight and height measurements evaluate the adequacy of local fat reserves, while the easier to measure mid-arm circumference assesses total growth of subcutaneous fat and muscle (Jelliffe, 1969). One problem is that anthropometric measures of heights and weights are usually age related and at the village level, ages are not usually reliably recorded. It is often more useful and accurate to evaluate weights against heights than to evaluate either height or weight with age related standards.

Death rates, especially infant mortality rates, are *indirect* indicators of nutritional and health problems but to be of value mortality rates must be assessed in the light of the local disease and infection pattern. Infant mortality rates can be obtained from local birth and death records and census data but these can be unreliable as not all infant deaths, especially those in the first few days of life, are recorded. Crude death rates, tuberculosis death rates and still birth rates are less common indicators.

Frequency of Different Methods in Village Surveys

The nutritional status of a population can be evaluated by food consumption data, physical data (anthropometric, clinical and biochemical) or both. To collect data on both physical measures of nutritional status and food consumption is obviously more costly. Even so, a higher proportion (48 per cent) of village nutrition surveys provide both types of data than either alone (see table 3.2). South East Asia is the exception: in India a high proportion of surveys provide only food consumption data while for the rest of Asia there are an equal proportion of surveys in each of the three categories (nutritional status surveys, food consumption surveys and physical status surveys). In the Middle East, very few surveys collect only food consumption data while six times as many provide data on physical measures of nutritional status. The only conclusive finding is that surveys providing only physical data are fewer in number than either 'food consumption' or 'nutritional status' surveys and that surveys collecting both food consumption and physical data (nutritional status surveys) predominate. We also found (table 4.1) that a higher proportion of food consumption surveys (47 per cent) have used the food weighment method which is more costly than all other food consumption survey methods except food composite analysis. Diet histories are next in popularity especially in Asia but these only provide qualitative information on food practices, taboos, etc. For all areas combined, a very high percentage of surveys (21 per cent) do not indicate what method was employed in the nutrition survey.

Comparative Methodologies

Ideally, choice of method should be determined by survey aims. But survey resources are not always unlimited and therefore choice of method will be restricted by available funds. It is important to weigh costs against reliability, asking how accurate results need to be, and what it will cost to increase accuracy in alternative ways; excessive costs incurred by large samples would often be better spent on field checks, supervision and re-interviewing. It is important to select

Table 4.1: Percentage of Village Food Consumption Surveys Using Different Types of Method

Area	Total Number of Surveys	Food Weighment	Food Composite Analysis	24-Hour Recall	Inventory Log Book Method	Seven-Day Record	Food Balance Sheet	Food Lists	Diet Histories	No Data
India	100	49	1	10	0	0	10	0	16	14
Africa	68	47.1	0	4.4	0	0	1.5	2.9	16.2	27.9
Latin America	54	48	1.9	3.7	1.9	0	0	0	16.7	27.8
Rest of Asia	26	19.2	3.8	7.7	0	3.8	0	0	46.2	19.2
Oceania	19	52.6	0	10.5	0	5.3	0	0	10.5	21.1
Middle East	14	71.4	7.1	0	0	0	0	0	7.1	14.3
Total	281	47	1.4	6.8	0.4	0.7	3.9	0.7	18.1	21

methods, however inflexibly, within the budget from the start: *ad hoc* adaptation of methods will give less reliable results.

For each survey, the relevant costs should include transport, labour, equipment and analysis but actual costs must include opportunity costs of alternative uses of the field worker, jeeps, equipment, etc. Size of sample, type of staff employed and length of survey are additional factors which add to the cost of the survey: the larger the sample the greater the cost but the smaller the error. Ideally the sample size should offer maximum accuracy within the limits of the money, personnel and time available but the key question is how much resources should be devoted to reduce sampling error. Nutritionists must be ready to advise on the acceptable margin: an error of plus or minus 5 per cent in nutrient consumption figures might be acceptable but an error of plus or minus 15 per cent might impair the practical value. In VSP's experience, much error-reducing effort spent on refining the sample would yield far more impact if concentrated on reducing non-sampling errors by training field-workers, by standardising and checking their methods and results, and by understanding the village background.

We should measure the trade-off between the benefits of a larger sample and those of (a) devoting more time to each person or household being assessed, (b) spending longer in establishing initial rapport or (c) reducing the number of field-workers. The costs of training, the hire of highly qualified personnel, field supervision, etc. should all be considered. Employment of highly qualified personnel will almost certainly add to the costs of the survey and qualifications are not always an advantage. Doctors tend to specialise in the diseases of the rich and may need re-training in order to recognise the specific clinical symptoms of deficiency diseases. But employment of unqualified personnel will require pre-field-work or even in-the-field training. Teachers are required for training, and afterwards supervision will be required in the field. But the cost of maintaining one supervisor per village may be prohibitive. Therefore, the cost of using untrained staff should be weighed against the additional costs of field supervision which are high but essential for any degree of standardisation in methods of measurement between survey staff.

All the above costs and alternatives should be taken into account. Then given a certain monetary allowance for the survey, the costs of different methods for fulfilling the survey aims should be evaluated in the above terms. The method giving the best chance of fulfilling the aims with respect to the provision of certain data requirements will be chosen bearing in mind the need to cost analysis and write-up. Thus the aims and data requirements of the survey will be constrained by both the practical costs of the survey and by the desired level of scientific accuracy.

The village surveys never indicate why methods are chosen: choice may have been determined by chance or by the qualification of the survey workers. We do not imply that survey costs are never evaluated but expensive methods were frequently undertaken and some surveys were left partially incomplete (from lack of funds?). Several surveys state, for example, that the method chosen was the seven-day weighment method but the qualitative results do not suggest this level of accuracy. In fact in some surveys, researchers apologise for incompleteness of data because monetary constraints became a problem half-way through the survey.

Comparison of methods employed in food consumption surveys can provide some useful guidelines as to choice of method. Such comparisons have already been made (see ICNND, 1962; Flores, 1965; Mahdavan and Swaminathan, 1966; Padmavati, 1958; Pasricha, 1959 and Périssé, 1968). In general, the food list method is cheap and quick but the inventory/log book method provides more data and demands less of the field-worker as the housewife weighs and records the food purchases. However, the housewife must be literate and the data obtained are still not as accurate as data obtained by food weighment. Since food composite analysis is expensive and time consuming the real choice of method for obtaining quantitative data is between recall and food weighment. The former is quicker because the amounts of foods consumed in the previous say 24 hours can easily be recorded at one interview whereas the weighment method involves weighing all meals (unless food is cooked once-a-day) and returning the following day to assess the amount of in-and-between meal eating. Both methods require trained investigators and extensive time for data calculation but unless food wastage, snacks between meals, seasonal intakes, physiological requirements and other factors are taken into account, then the degree of reliability obtained by more expensive and time consuming methods may not justify the extra cost.

Recall methods are more accurate if they use standardised vessels for estimating the volume of foods consumed. In that case, the errors of food weighment must be kept to a minimum in order to obtain results significantly more reliable than the 24-hour recall method. If resources are limited and investigators are determined to weigh rather than rely on recall, then either we reduce the sample size or weigh over three days rather than the usual seven. However, a shorter period is probably not advisable, because almost all cultures feature a weekly holiday or holy day, on which food consumption behaviour takes special forms. If known, however, this might be allowed for. A high research priority, on the evidence we have seen, should go to efforts to test the reliability and costs of periodic weighment — say for four days selected at random throughout the seasons. Especially in a centre carrying out many rotating studies, a major saving in costs might be possible. Alternatively, a given outlay might provide more reliable results if used to make field checks than if used to extend the number of 'weighing' days. If data reliability is a high priority relative to economy, the weighment method should be chosen since it is invaluable for providing reliable data on intra-household and inter-household distribution of foods, preferably over time. Food consumption surveys should be flexible: if intensive pilot surveys indicate that PCM is the main and most widespread deficiency problem and that certain foods are the main protein and calorie sources, future surveys could concentrate on measuring the consumption of these foods instead of the entire diet. Similarly, in order to comprehend the nutritional status of the total village, we may in future be able to limit our survey to certain sectors (Blankhart, 1971).

Food consumption surveys are costly and must not be employed if other, cheaper methods will do instead. At a given survey cost it may be better to be 95 per cent sure of the nutritional problems in five regions, than 99 per cent sure — via weighment — of the problems of one. Once the problem has been located, the fastest and cheapest method for measuring the extent of malnutrition in the population as a whole must be determined. For certain diagnoses such as the severity and incidence of anaemia, clinical examinations are cheaper and give results more quickly. Clinical examination is most useful where symptoms can be assigned to specific causes (e.g. goitre is a specific sign of iodine deficiency). But as clinical examinations identify extreme rather than moderate cases of malnutrition they should be employed as a screening procedure. The incidence of oedema could, for example, be used as a 'public health index of nutritional status' (Bailey, 1962, p. 10). The main problem with clinical assessment is that long periods of deficiency occur before clinical symptoms appear. For an up-to-date assessment of the situation, biochemical studies are more accurate as they provide information on nutrient intake and adequacy at the time of the survey. However, they are expensive and if the results of the clinical survey indicate severe and widespread anaemia it may be cheaper and more sensible to implement the programme on these results alone than to instigate biochemical studies which are an additional expense. Unless of course a quick assay of, for example, the blood albumen level (Collis, 1962) could indicate the nutritional status of the population. Even then, costs of sample analysis are still high.

Anthropometric data can be easily and simply collected to provide measures of growth status and protein calorie malnutrition. There is also less variation in the standardisation of data between surveys and between investigators than for clinical surveys. Choice of data will depend on the subject. Heights and weights are useful indicators in age groups where growth should be steadily increasing whereas skinfold thicknesses are a good measure of the effect of seasonal hunger on the adult male work-force population. Anthropometric measurements are probably the best indicators of the benefits of nutrition programmes aimed at pre-school and school children, though a carefully selected control group is essential if the effects of such a scheme are to be separated from those of other contemporaneous changes, and the scheme's nutritional benefit accurately calculated.

Conclusions

Several methods are available for the measurement of village nutritional status but the most frequently used method, food weighment, was, for some lines of enquiry the most expensive. For cheaper evaluation, and collection of food consumption data we would support the extended use of other methods (24-hour recall). Clinical surveys need to be conducted with care but their main value lies in indicating potential areas of poor nutrition for future survey work. Anthropometric data are useful measures of nutritional status on their own or with other types of data, and also have a wide potential use for the evaluation of the effect of applied nutrition programmes. Collecting biochemical data on subsamples of a larger survey population may provide important information but runs into problems of high cost, transportation of samples, laboratory standardisation and difficulties in drawing blood from wary villagers. Indirect data (vital statistics) at best vaguely indicate possible problem areas.

The costs and benefits of each method should be, but often are not, adequately considered at the beginning of each survey. Given the survey aims and implicitly the data to be obtained, one should first find out what type of methods are practical within certain cost limits. Second, one should select the method which will give the most relevant and accurate data within the budget. Unfortunately, there is little information on survey costs. The results of many surveys seemed less reliable than one would expect if finance had in fact been available to complete the method described. Reports rarely discussed monetary constraints.

Research is needed to evaluate survey methods, to compare the reliability and value of data collected by different methods, and at different levels of cost. It would be useful for policy planners and nutritionists if a manual could be prepared, showing how to calculate the costs of different methods of collecting data. This should provide a detailed breakdown of the costs of implementation under various conditions depending on length of residence in the village, size of survey team, sample size, etc. Research personnel are not *ipso facto* financial planners or fund raisers and it is therefore desirable that they have access to an appropriate specialist (an accountant or financial planner). Methods of field-work training should also be standardised in and between institutions but one practical consideration in terms of professional resources and costs will be the development of methods which can be used by relatively untrained and inexperienced interviewers. Research is required to improve methods of data collection, to standardise existing techniques and to improve methods for the collection of socio-economic data on the causes of poor nutrition which will provide a better basis for improvement than proximate data alone. We need to evaluate to what extent the nutritional level of populations can be ascertained from measuring the nutritional status of certain age groups and know what types of nutrition data to collect in conjunction with other sorts of surveys.

5 INTER-VILLAGE DIFFERENCES IN NUTRITION AND VILLAGE CLASSIFICATION BY TYPE OF DIET

The data bank for the VSP nutrition research consists of 360 nutrition oriented surveys which provide data for about 900 villages in the less developed world. Analysis of these studies showed that 'ultimate' data on the key village socio-economic characteristics are poor. 'Proximate' data on the size and type of nutritional problem are more frequent and constitute the bulk of the data. We were unable to identify the whole range of factors affecting village diets or to be sure that the variables we have selected are the key variables. However, rather than waste this 'never before collected or used' bank of village nutrition data, we attempted to fulfil the primary aims of the programme and identify types of village diet by using mainly this proximate data with a minimum amount of socio-economic information. Our village classification is by:

1. Village Ecology
2. Type of Main Food Staple
3. Village Economy
4. Value of Food Consumption
5. Village Location and Accessibility

The data on which this analysis is based are second-hand and extracted from a non-random selection of village studies. Therefore the typology is not comprehensive or statistically representative but at least demonstrates the type of approach to the identification of micro-level problems that we in the VSP are advocating.

Classification by Village Ecology

In subsistence villages, the type of diet is in part determined by ecological factors of which climate is one factor affecting cropping patterns, productivity and therefore the availability of food throughout the year. Isolation of climate as the key ecological variable is somewhat arbitrary to say the least but some of our results are significant and our general theory, which at the subsistence level has been supported by numerous observations from field-workers, is that villages with a unimodal distribution of rain, no irrigation and one annual harvest will rely on post-harvest food supplies which determine the size and distribution of village calories not just at the time, but until the next harvest. Seasonal food shortages are common as on-farm grain stocks are running low before the next harvest. The only alternative is to buy food but prices are high at this time until pulled down by the impending harvest. Only the existence of adequate storage can facilitate the adequate distribution of food over the year (i.e. even if enough is produced to feed the village until the next harvest) but still there are no guarantees. Villages with continuous cropping or staggered multiple cropping patterns with either irrigation or a bimodal distribution of rain might be better off throughout the year and can obviate the need for storage facilities.

We tried to examine nutritional differences between seasons. We expected to find an adequate supply of food in the dry season after the harvest and poorer supplies in the wet season when harvest stocks are running low. Analysis of the 360 nutrition-specific surveys showed that even proximate data providing evidence on the size and type of nutrition problem by season was limited. Fifteen per cent of village specific nutrition surveys from the less developed world provide data on seasonal nutrition. Twenty-nine of these are from Africa and comprise five Nigerian villages, one from Ghana, eight from the Cameroons, five Senegalese villages, five from the Ivory Coast and five from Togo. In comparison, only two Indian surveys provide data on seasonal food consumption.

In a non-random sample of 25 African villages with information on seasonal nutrition, the agricultural year was divided into a dry period and a wet season. In our analysis, the differences in calorie intakes, requirements and the percentage fulfilment of requirements were evaluated between and within seasons using a 't' test. A significant difference (at 1 per cent) was found between the percentage fulfilment of calorie requirements in the wet (85 per cent) and dry (92 per cent) seasons. This was related to mildly significant (at 10 per cent) differences in calorie intakes but not in requirements. These are not usually adjusted for seasonal differences in labour inputs and anyhow usually include the requirements for the non-work-force section of the population. Assuming one-third of the population works in the wet season, the net effect of their additional requirements will result in a small increase in requirements for the total population. We found that only seven more calories per person per day were needed in the wet season which is surprising in view of the additional energy requirements. The larger calorie intakes in the dry season (2,102 calories per person per day compared with 1,885 calories per person per day in the wet season) might reflect a higher consumption level of food staples abundant in the post-harvest period.

A further analysis was conducted on the sample differentiated on the basis of rainfall modality. Villages with a bimodal distribution of rain have less seasonal variation in their diets because there is a greater probability that there will be two annual harvests rather than one which will provide for the more equal distribution of foods throughout the year. Where annual food availability depends on the productivity of one harvest, food shortages are more likely to occur and because of the exponential growth of pest population and damage in confined space (Lipton, 1968) a one harvest system throws a greater strain upon food storage facilities. In the 15 villages with a unimodal rainy season, the percentage fulfilment of calorie requirements was 100 per cent in the dry season and 88 per cent in the wet season; the difference between seasons is significant at 0.5 per cent, and reflects differences in intake (2,191 calories *per capita* per day in the wet season compared with 2,458 in the dry) rather than requirement levels. The difference between calorie intakes independent of requirements in the wet and dry season is more significant in villages with one period of rainfall (although only at the 10 per cent level) than in villages with two rainy seasons. Multi-cropping villages with a unimodal rainfall did not meet calorie requirements in either season; the gap between seasons was around 10 per cent. Single crop villages with a unimodal distribution of rain met calorie requirements only in the dry season and inter-seasonal differences in the percentage fulfilment of calorie requirements were 13 per cent. For villages with a bimodal distribution of rain the differences between the percentage fulfilment of calorie requirements in the wet and dry seasons were not significantly different. Thus, *between* villages, our African data suggest that those villages located in climatic zones where the rain supply is unimodal, irrigation is absent and storage facilities are inadequate, are at most risk of seasonal food shortages. Within these broad ecological zones, more village types characterised by other socio-economic variables may be identifiable.

Classification by Type of Main Food Staple

We hypothesise that in rural areas: (1) cropping patterns, culturally determined food habits, food preferences and purchasing patterns provide for a monotonous diet; and that (2) as food staples constitute the bulk of the diet and are consumed in such large quantities, deficiencies characteristic of these main staples may also typify the entire diet. For example, certain food staples are characteristically deficient in some nutrients: maize is deficient in niacin (FAO, 1953) and white rice in thiamine (FAO, 1964). Although comparative studies of diets based on different staples are few (those by Nicol, 1959 and Périssé, 1962 being two of the few exceptions) their evidence suggested that we might be able to group village diets by type of main food staple. For example, Nicol found that protein intakes and scores were higher in the cereal based diets (sorghum and millet based diet) than in the yam eating areas 'where the diets supplied a little more than the minimum protein requirement, but they never provided the safe practical allowance' (Nicol, 1959, p. 313). These were the sorts of results we tested for.

We identified the main staple as the food contributing the largest number of calories. Diets with several staples were ignored and data from only those villages where the staple could be clearly identified were used. Five main staples were found: cassava, millet, potato, rice and maize. Unfortunately, our material permitted us to establish only three sample populations. We were forced to aggregate data for (1) all African countries and (2) all Latin American countries. Too few village data from other continents were available for reliable statistical analysis. However, villages characterised by the same food staples from Africa, Latin America and South East Asia were also combined to provide what we have called (3) the 'world' sample.

We used *discriminate analysis* to measure the statistical reliability of classifying villages by their main food staple as cassava villages, millet, potato, rice or maize villages. We identified the main food staple in the diet of each village and 'forecast' that each village would be allocated to its corresponding group in the discriminate analysis test on the basis of other variables measuring diet adequacy. We were limited by our data in the number and types of variables we could choose. The discriminate analysis test was conducted twice on each sample using different classifactory variables. Test 1 variables included, for each village, the intake levels of calories, protein, calcium, iron, Vitamin A, thiamine, riboflavin, niacin and Vitamin C. Test 2 was based on figures for the adequacy of each of these nutrients in the diet of each village.

Discriminate analysis measures (a) the probability of allocating each village to a group other than that forecast: for example, whether each cassava village demonstrates the pattern of nutrient intake or adequacy of this group or has more in common with another group such as maize; (b) whether all the groups are significantly different from each other (Rao's F test and Bartlett's Chi-squared test) and (c) whether pairs of village types such as millet vs. maize are significantly different (Mahalanobis' D-squared test). The final results of both tests 1 and 2 are presented for each sample in a 'Hits and Misses' table (for an example see table 5.2, p. 59). In this test, each village forecast by type of main staple to belong to a group is allocated on the basis of its dietary characteristics, nutrient intake in test 1 and nutrient adequacy in test 2, to its actual group. The *total forecast group membership* figure denotes the number of villages of the type of main staple which is named at the head of each *column*. The *total actual group membership* figure in each *row* denotes the actual membership of each group as measured by the discriminate analysis test. We can then calculate the

percentage of villages displaced from their forecast group (defined by
their main staple) into their actual groups and therefore how reliable
and useful our classification of village diets by type of main staple
actually is.

There are obvious weaknesses in this analysis: the sample is biased,
consisting of a non-random selection of only those villages for which
the data was most adequate. The available data also usually ignore
(a) inter-village differences in demographic structure which affect
requirements and (b) to a great extent, seasonal differences in food
consumption. The most serious objection to this approach is that even
if we succeed in classifying village diets by type of main staple, this
may not be the key variable. Lack of socio-economic data prevented
an evaluation of the types of features common to villages with the same
food staple. Another problem lies in the analysis. Intake levels of
nutrients were calculated from food composition tables, and largely
reflect intakes of those nutrients in the staple, which is also the basis
of the forecast of the discriminate analysis. If villagers ate only the
main food staple, each village would obviously fall into its forecast
group. So what the discriminate analysis measures must be the extent
to which other foods cancel out the differences in the nutrient
adequacy of the main food staple. For the supplementation of diets
it is important to know whether this nutrient compensation or levelling
is occurring. In spite of these drawbacks, this type of nutritional
classification has never — to our knowledge — been conducted and
could prove a useful example as a potential tool for research workers
attempting a nation-wide or even regional survey where primary data
have to be collected.

Results of the Discriminate Analysis Test 1 Based on Nutrient Intake Data

For the Latin American sample of villages, sufficient data were available
for the identification of only three village types: maize, potato and rice.
The diets of the three groups (as measured by the pattern of nutrient
intake) were found to be significantly different at the 0.1 per cent level
but between individual groups, significant differences were only found
between maize and rice diets (at the 5 per cent level) and between
maize and potato diets at the 0.1 per cent level. Differences between
potato and rice diets were not found to be significant which indicates
that maize diets have features which distinguish them from both potato
and rice diets.

Table 5.1 provides data on the mean nutrient intakes of each village
type in the Latin American sample. Intakes of calories, protein,
thiamine and riboflavin were very similar but intakes of calcium and
Vitamins A and C were more disparate. If we compare differences in

Table 5.1: Results of the Discriminate Analysis Test 1 — Mean Nutrient Intakes

Area	Village Type	N	Calories	Protein (g)	Calcium (mg)	Iron (mg)	Vitamin A (IU)	Thiamine (mg)	Riboflavin (mg)	Niacin (mg)	Vitamin C (mg)
Latin America	Maize	30	2010	56.3	782	17.3	1254	1.6	0.8	15.4	44.8
	Potatoes	9	2100	57.7	447	22.3	2403	1.2	0.99	22.4	109
	Rice	4	1823	54.3	346	12.3	4485	1.1	0.9	11.7	83.6
Africa	Cassava	17	1893	42.5	460	13.2	7346	0.9	0.6	11.4	162.9
	Millet	6	1990	63.8	419	16.3	2397	1.8	0.9	15	31
World	Maize	31	2029	57.5	767	17.6	1223	1.6	0.8	15.4	44.1
	Potatoes	9	2100	57.7	447	22.3	2403	1.2	0.99	22.4	109
	Rice	8	1828	53.8	320	13.8	8908	1.2	0.7	11.2	60.8
	Millet	6	1990	63.8	419	16.3	2397	1.8	0.9	15	31
	Cassava	17	1893	42.5	460	13.2	7346	0.9	0.6	11.4	162.9

nutrient intakes between these villages we see that the calcium intakes in maize diets are notably high while intakes of Vitamin C are relatively low. However, intra-group variations in intakes of calcium and Vitamin A are high and the F ratio indicates that niacin, Vitamin C, iron and Vitamin A have a greater effect (in that order) on inter-group dietary differences than any other nutrient. With such a small sample it is obviously difficult to draw reliable conclusions from this test but the results are interesting in view of the fact that niacin deficits are a common feature of maize diets and that potatoes are the only one of these three staples to provide Vitamin C.

The 'Hits and Misses' table 5.2 shows that out of a total of 43 villages forecast to belong to their main food staple group, only three (6 per cent) were reallocated in the discriminate analysis test to other groups. This is an extremely small number and indicates that for this non-random sample of villages we have discriminated between types of village diet characterised by main staple. It is interesting to note that none of the potato villages which are all located in one small area of Ecuador have been reallocated to another group.

For the African village sample three village types were identified: cassava, millet and maize. The maize group was omitted from the test because the sample was too small. The diets of cassava and millet villages, as measured by the nutrient intakes of calories, protein, calcium, iron, Vitamin A, thiamine, riboflavin, niacin and Vitamin C, were found to be significantly different at the 1 per cent level by Bartlett's Chi-squared test and at the 2.5 per cent level by Rao's F test and Mahalanobis' D-squared test.

Table 5.1 indicates that differences in nutrient intakes between the two groups were highest for Vitamin C, Vitamin A, thiamine and protein. Intra-group variations in intake were high for Vitamin A and thiamine while the F ratio indicates that the most important variables distinguishing cassava diets from millet were protein and Vitamin C intakes. Since cassava is a poor protein source and richer in Vitamin C than millet, these results corroborate our hypotheses although Vitamin C can be destroyed in the preparation process.

The 'Hits and Misses' table 5.3 shows that out of a total of 23 villages only one (4 per cent) village forecast as a cassava village was reallocated to the millet group. This village had extremely low intake levels of Vitamins A and C and a higher protein intake in comparison with the mean figures for the cassava group.

Combining the same village types from Latin America, Africa and South East Asia provided us with five groups for the *World* sample: maize, potato, rice, millet and cassava. Differences in nutrient intakes between the five groups were significant at the 0.1 per cent level but between individual groups, significant differences were only found

Table 5.2: 'Hits and Misses' Table for the Sample of Latin American Villages Based on Nutrient Intake Data (Test 1)

		Columns		
		Maize	Potato	Rice	Total Actual Group Membership
Rows	Maize	28	0	1	29
	Potato	0	9	0	9
	Rice	2	0	3	5
	Total forecast group member-ship	30	9	4	43

between maize and cassava diets (at the 0.1 per cent level) and between maize and potato villages at the 5 per cent level.

Table 5.1 indicates that protein intakes were lowest and Vitamin C intakes highest in cassava villages. However, the test shows that cassava and maize diets are distinguishable by differences in intakes of Vitamins A, C, thiamine and calcium. Differences between maize and potato diets are distinguishable by intakes of Vitamins C, A and calcium. For all groups combined, the F ratio indicates that intake levels of Vitamin C and niacin are, in that order, the main determinants of dietary differences between the five types of diets.

The 'Hits and Misses' table 5.4 shows that out of a total of 71 villages, 10 (14 per cent) were removed from their forecast group (measured by main staple) to other groups with more similar dietary characteristics. These reallocations were highest (50 per cent) for rice villages which is not really surprising as these rice villages have been taken from widely different continents (Africa, Latin America, India and South East Asia). No potato villages were replaced which again indicates that this type of analysis is far more reliable for measuring intra-country variations in dietary types.

Results of the Discriminate Analysis Test 2 Based on Nutrient Adequacy (Percentage Fulfilment of Nutrient Requirements)

More surveys provide data on nutrient adequacy of village diets than on mean nutrient intakes. Thus village samples for tests 1 and 2 are not comparable: a few villages have been added to test 1 samples and some removed to provide test 2 samples. To calculate their adequacy, the mean nutrient intakes for either the entire village or a representative sample are calculated and presented as a percentage of the nutrient requirements for that population which were specified in the study.

Table 5.3: 'Hits and Misses' Table for the Sample of African Villages Based on Nutrient Intake Data (Test 1)

		Columns		
		Cassava	Millet	Total Actual Group Membership
Rows	Cassava	16	0	16
	Millet	1	6	7
	Total forecast group membership	17	6	23

The same three types of village were identified for the Latin American sample: maize, potato and rice. Results similar to those of test 1 were obtained: differences between the three groups were significant at the 0.1 per cent level but only differences between maize and potato and between maize and rice villages were significant at the 0.1 and 1 per cent levels, respectively. Differences between potato and rice villages were not — as in the other test — found to be significant.

Differences in nutrient adequacy between maize and potato diets are greatest for calcium, niacin and Vitamin C (see table 5.5). Similar differences were observed in test 1. Between maize and rice diets, differences in the adequacy of Vitamins A and C and calcium were forecast. As in the first test the dietary adequacy of calcium and Vitamin C seem to be the distinguishing feature of maize diets although the F ratio indicates that the adequacy of niacin, Vitamin A and iron are, in that order, the features that distinguish these diets from each other.

The 'Hits and Misses' table 5.6 shows that out of a total of 44 villages, only two (4.5 per cent) were reallocated during the test: one of these was from the maize group (reallocated to the potato group) and one was in the rice group (reallocated to the maize group). As in the other test, no potato villages were reallocated.

Cassava, millet and maize villages were identified for the African sample. Differences between the three groups were found to be significant at the 2.5 per cent level but the differences between cassava and the other dietary types were greater than differences between millet and maize diets especially in the adequacy of thiamine, riboflavin, Vitamins A and C (see table 5.5). Cassava diets are characteristically deficient in protein with surpluses of Vitamins A and C. The 'Hits and Misses' table 5.7 (p. 64) shows that relatively few cassava villages were reallocated to other groups; 25 per cent of the total

Table 5.4: 'Hits and Misses' Table for the 'World' Sample of Village Types Based on Nutrient Intake Data (Test 1)

		Columns					
		Maize	Potatoes	Rice	Millet	Cassava	Total Actual Group Membership
	Maize	28	0	3	1	2	34
	Potatoes	0	9	0	0	0	9
	Rice	0	0	4	0	0	4
Rows	Millet	1	0	0	5	0	6
	Cassava	2	0	1	0	15	18
	Total fore-cast group membership	31	9	8	6	17	71

number of villages were reallocated to groups other than their forecast groups.

Villages of the same type from Latin America, Africa and South East Asia were combined to provide a 'world' sample of five village types. Differences between all the groups are significant at 0.1 per cent (Rao's F test and Bartlett's Chi-squared test) but significant differences were only found between cassava and maize (at the 0.1 per cent level), potatoes and maize (at the 1 per cent level) and between rice and maize (at the 5 per cent level). Thus all diets except millet are significantly different from maize diets. If we exclude millet diets from the comparison, we find that in maize diets, intakes of Vitamins A and C are low and intakes of thiamine and calcium are high relative to the intakes of those nutrients in cassava, potato and rice diets. The F ratio, however, indicates that between these dietary types niacin intakes followed by Vitamin C, thiamine and calcium are the distinguishing variables.

The 'Hits and Misses' table 5.8 (p. 65) shows that out of a total of 90 villages, 25 per cent were reallocated to new groups. The largest number of reallocations were in the millet group (57 per cent), followed by rice (35 per cent), cassava (30 per cent) and maize (20 per cent).

Classification by Village Economy

Because of the danger of cultivating cash crops at the expense of subsistence crops in terms of land, labour and equipment, and of not spending the money received from crop sales to nutritional advantage, cash crop villages are often nutritionally worse off than villages growing and consuming their own products. Evidence shows (Périssé,

Table 5.5: Results of the Discriminate Analysis Test 2 Based on Nutrient Adequacy (Mean Percentage Fulfilment of Nutrient Requirements)

Area	Village Type	N	Calories	Protein	Calcium	Iron	Vitamin A	Thiamine	Riboflavin	Niacin	Vitamin C
Latin America	Maize	31	90.4	93.5	113.4	156.5	46.8	136.1	49.9	108.2	84
	Potato	9	96.8	93.9	44.9	200.7	55.6	105.1	64.9	205.3	157.4
	Rice	4	82	97	56	112.5	133.8	102	54	80.5	154.3
Africa	Cassava	20	86.2	73	50.6	131.7	173.7	74.7	36.1	92.8	292.6
	Millet	7	88.1	94.3	57.6	137.9	51.7	152.4	76.1	126.4	24.4
	Maize	9	83.2	98.4	38.8	132.6	32.2	203.4	79.9	143.1	147.1
World	Cassava	20	86.2	73	50.6	131.7	168.6	74.7	36.1	92.8	292.6
	Millet	7	88.1	94.3	57.6	137.9	51.7	152.4	76.1	126.4	69.6
	Potato	9	96.8	93.9	44.9	200.7	55.6	105.1	64.9	205.3	157.4
	Rice	14	81.6	85.8	51.3	115.4	129.9	95.7	39.4	84.2	173.8
	Maize	40	88.8	94.6	96.6	151.1	43.6	153.3	56.7	116	98.3

Table 5.6: 'Hits and Misses' Table for the Sample of Latin American Villages Based on the Adequacy of Different Nutrients in the Diet (Test 2)

		Columns			
		Maize	Potato	Rice	Total Actual Group Membership
Rows	Maize	30	0	1	31
	Potato	1	9	0	10
	Rice	0	0	3	3
	Total forecast group membership	31	9	4	44

1962) that subsistence crops (e.g. groundnuts) which are increasingly sold for cash gradually get omitted from the diet. Other evidence from three Congolese villages showed that thiamine and niacin deficiencies occurred or were more serious in the village where all the groundnut crop was sold than in the villages where 'la plus grande partie est consomme sur place' (Ministère de la Cooperation, 1967, p. 182). Similarly, incentives to increase milk production for sale in nearby urban markets efficiently removed one of the main sources of animal protein from an Indian village (Jyothi, 1963).

As the importance of cash crops increases so may their cultivated area increase at the expense of the acreage devoted to subsistence crops (Collis, 1962) or the cash crop (cocoa) can shade the ground so that nothing else will grow there. Food crops which are easy to grow and quick to cook (cassava) often replace traditional crops as more time and energy is spent on the cultivation of cash crops. Unfortunately, these 'easy-to-grow' crops are often of poor nutritional value (Tanzanian National Nutrition Unit, n.d., p. 33). Returns from cash crops are not always immediate and if credit facilities are poor or nonexistent, cash to care for these crops must be obtained elsewhere, sometimes at the expense of food crops as in the Nigerian village of Ijana Itarua where 'families have much younger cocoa which has to be cared for with cash from the sale of their food crops' (Collis and others, 1962b, p. 208). Villages with a higher acreage of cash crops than subsistence crops will obviously spend a higher percentage of their income on food but scarcity of subsistence crops is not always compensated for by extra cash income as this is often channelled into the non-food sectors of the household budget or is spent all-in-one-go on expensive and luxurious foods. Thus Collis argues that

Table 5.7: 'Hits and Misses' Table for the Sample of African Villages
Based on the Adequacy of Different Nutrients in the Diet (Test 2)

		Columns			
		Cassava	Millet	Maize	Total Actual Group Membership
Rows	Cassava	17	0	2	19
	Millet	1	5	1	7
	Maize	2	2	6	10
	Total forecast group member-ship	20	7	9	36

Cocoa is one of the best cash crops in the world, giving the highest yield for the smallest energy output. One might then expect the cocoa villagers to be well off, well fed, happy and gay. We found exactly the reverse. The people were dull, apathetic and unhappy. Their villages were run down, dirty and dilapidated and their children naked, pot-bellied and sickly. The reason for this is that it is not enough to introduce a highly paying cash crop to an illiterate peasantry and expect them to profit by it. What happens is that it tends to kill their traditional life, merely putting money in their pockets for a short period in the year, during which time they enjoy themselves. When the money gets scarce, months before the next harvest, they find themselves short of everything. [Collis, 1962b, p. 223]

In order to spot any nutritional differences between cash crop and subsistence villages we took a non-random selection of villages from Africa and Latin America. Villages were classified into one of three economic groups: (1) *Pure Subsistence villages* which produce almost all the food they consume and neither market nor purchase major amounts of crops or foods; (2) *Semi-Subsistence villages* which sell part of their subsistence food crop and purchase food with either this income or alternative sources such as wage earning and (3) *Semi-Cash crop villages* which produce both cash and subsistence crops, marketing either or both and buy some but not all of their food. We define cash crops as those products which are either (a) non-edible, e.g. cotton, (b) an unimportant nutrient source, e.g. tobacco, or are (c) not usually included in large quantities or totally absent from the subsistence diet, e.g. cocoa.

Again we used discriminate analysis to measure the statistical reliability of classifying diets by type of village economy in Africa, Latin

Table 5.8: 'Hits and Misses' Table for the 'World' Sample of Village Types Based on Nutrient Adequacy (Test 2)

		Columns					
		Cassava	Millet	Potatoes	Rice	Maize	Total Actual Group Membership
	Cassava	14	0	0	4	2	20
	Millet	0	3	0	0	0	3
	Potatoes	0	0	9	0	0	9
Rows	Rice	5	0	0	9	6	20
	Maize	1	4	0	1	32	38
	Total forecast group membership	20	7	9	14	40	90

America and in a combined 'world' sample. The test was conducted twice on each sample using different classificatory variables. Test A variables included, for each village, the intake levels of calories, protein, calcium, iron, Vitamin A, thiamine, riboflavin, niacin and Vitamin C. Test B was based on figures for the adequacy of each of these nutrients in the diet of each village.

Results of the Discriminate Analysis Test A Based on Nutrient Intake Data

We were able to group 33 Latin American villages by type of economy but unfortunately dietary differences based on nutrient intakes between the three groups were not found to be significant. The 'Hits and Misses' table 5.10 shows that as many as 27 per cent of all the villages forecast to belong to one particular economic group were reallocated to other groups during the test.

For the African sample, 29 villages were identifiable by 'type of economy'. Dietary differences between pure-subsistence, semi-subsistence and semi-cash crop villages were found to be significant at 0.1 per cent (Bartlett's Chi-squared test) and 1 per cent (Rao's F test). Table 5.9 shows that there is a great deal of inter-group variation in nutrient intakes but that these levels are generally higher (with the exception of Vitamins A and C) in pure-subsistence villages than any other type. The F ratio indicates that intakes of protein, iron and calcium are, in that order, the variables which distinguish these diets from each other.

The 'Hits and Misses' table 5.11 shows that out of a total of 29 villages forecast to belong to an economic group, only two were reallocated in the discriminate analysis test to other groups.

Table 5.9: Results of the Discriminate Analysis Test A (Mean Nutrient Intakes)

Area	Village type	N	Calories	Protein (g)	Calcium (mg)	Iron (mg)	Vitamin A (IU)	Thiamine (mg)	Riboflavin (mg)	Niacin (mg)	Vitamin C (mg)
Latin America	Pure	4	1680	51.8	601	16.4	1697	1.6	0.6	12.4	43.8
	Semi-subsistence	18	1993	54	729	19.5	2503	1.4	0.9	17.5	74.1
	Semi-cash crop	11	1983	51.7	658	16.2	1938	1.4	0.7	15.8	50
Africa	Pure	8	2219	78.5	1206	29.3	4533	4	0.9	16.7	64.3
	Semi-subsistence	7	1802	45	488	14.9	2967	1.2	0.6	11.8	68.7
	Semi-cash crop	14	1870	44.8	438	17.1	7623	1.2	0.7	13.4	153.9
Combined sample	Pure	12	2040	69.6	1004	25	3588	3.2	0.8	15.3	57.5
	Semi-subsistence	25	1939	51.5	661	18.2	2633	1.34	0.8	15.9	72.6
	Semi-cash crop	25	1920	47.8	535	16.7	5122	1.3	0.7	7.7	108.2

Table 5.10: 'Hits and Misses' Table for the Sample of Latin American Villages Based on Nutrient Intake Data (Test A)

		Columns		
		Pure Subsistence	Semi-Subsistence	Semi-Cash Crop	Total Actual Group Membership
Rows	Pure subsistence	2	0	0	2
	Semi-subsistence	1	13	2	16
	Semi-cash crop	1	5	9	15
	Total forecast group membership	4	18	11	33

Amalgamation of the same village types from Latin America and Africa provided a 'world' sample of 62 villages. The discriminate analysis test revealed that for this sample, dietary differences between the three village types were significant at the 0.1 per cent level (Bartlett's Chi-squared test). With the exception of a few nutrients (notably Vitamins A and C) nutrient intake levels were higher in the pure subsistence villages and lowest in the semi-cash crop villages. The implication is that pure subsistence villages are better fed than villages which perhaps oversell their subsistence crops or cultivate cash crops at the expense of subsistence crops. We cannot substantiate these conclusions because we do not have sufficient data on crop production, size of sales or expenditure patterns for all those villages and therefore cannot identify the socio-economic factors responsible for differences in the diets of these village types.

The F ratio indicates that intakes of protein, iron and calcium are, in that order, the variables which distinguish these dietary types. However, the 'Hits and Misses' table 5.12 shows that despite significant differences between them, a high percentage (39 per cent) of villages are reallocated to groups other than their forecast ones.

Results of the Discriminate Analysis Test B Based on Nutrient Adequacy (Percentage Fulfilment of Nutrient Requirements)

Villages were classified by type of economy and their diets described in terms of nutrient adequacy. Discriminate analysis was conducted on a sample of African and Latin American villages and on a combined 'world' sample of villages from both areas. Differences between these dietary types were not found to be significant.

Classification by Expenditure on Food as a Percentage of Total Expenditure

Although we have argued that many villages in less developed countries produce most of the foods they consume, there are some that either

Table 5.11: 'Hits and Misses' Table for the Sample of African Villages Based on Nutrient Intake Data (Test A)

| | | Columns | | | |
		Pure Subsistence	Semi-Subsistence	Semi-Cash Crop	Total Actual Group Membership
	Pure subsistence	7	0	0	7
	Semi-subsistence	1	7	1	9
Rows	Semi-cash crop	0	0	13	13
	Total forecast group membership	8	7	14	29

purchase most of the food they need or purchase at least a few foods. For 22 African villages with data on expenditure, the mean food expenditure as a percentage of total expenditure was 48 per cent with a range of 9 to 80 per cent depending on subsistence productivity, income levels and purchasing patterns. Total food expenditure is high in villages of poor subsistence production, land shortages and high incomes. Village data indicate that food expenditure increases as income levels rise but when expressed as a percentage of total expenditure, decrease at higher income levels (Subramanian, 1964 and Nair, 1961).

However, high income villages with a low expenditure on food as a percentage of total expenditure are not necessarily nutritionally better off than low income villages with a high proportion of their total expenditure spent on food: subsistence productivity must also be taken into account. For this reason data on total food expenditure alone is not a useful measure of village nutritional status. We therefore extracted data on the monetary value of total food consumption from a non-random selection of villages from all over India and correlated these figures with socio-economic data. These villages were surveyed by the Indian Census (Delhi and Rajasthan) and by the following Agro-Economic Research Centres (AERCs): Delhi, Madhya Pradesh, Sardar Patel, Uttar Pradesh, Madras and Visva Bharati. The Delhi Centre surveys villages in Uttar Pradesh, Punjab, Haryana and Himachal Pradesh; Sardar Patel covers Gujarat and Rajasthan; the Uttar Pradesh AERC surveys villages in Uttar Pradesh, Punjab and Haryana; Madras AERC covers Tamil Nadu, Mysore, Kerala and Andra Pradesh and the Visva Bharati AERC surveys villages in West Bengal, Bihar and Orissa. Unfortunately, these data were too poor and too varied to calculate the nutrient adequacy of these diets and we could only correlate socio-economic data with the value and not the quantity of foods consumed. Data on the value of food consumption were collected by

Table 5.12: 'Hits and Misses' Table for the 'World' Sample of Village Types Based on Nutrient Intake Data (Test A)

		Columns			
		Pure Subsistence	Semi-Subsistence	Semi-Cash Crop	Total Actual Group Membership
	Pure subsistence	8	1	1	10
	Semi-subsistence	4	20	14	38
Rows	Semi-cash crops	0	4	10	14
	Total forecast group membership	12	25	25	62

different methods and the results are often aggregated for food groups such as cereals and pulses. Food value data includes (1) the total value (rupees) of cereals and pulses consumed per household; (2) the total value of cereal and pulse consumption as a percentage of the total value of food consumption; (3) the value of total food consumption as a percentage of total expenditure; (4) the value of wheat and rice consumption as a percentage of the total value of food consumption, and (5) the value of millet consumption as a percentage of the value of total consumption.

The results (table 5.13) show a wide range of food consumption values: the value of total food consumption as a percentage of total expenditure ranges from 55 per cent (Delhi) to 78 per cent (Visva Bharati). This percentage is lowest where the total value of cereal and pulse consumption is highest (Rs 891/−) but where cereal and pulse consumption is a low percentage (31 per cent) of the total value of food consumed, which suggests high incomes for the villages surveyed by the Delhi AERC in the Punjab and Haryana which are relatively better off (high income levels) than other villages surveyed by the AERCs. Value of cereal and pulse consumption is also high for the Uttar Pradesh AERC whose sample includes the relatively richer villages of the Punjab and Haryana. Total value of cereal and pulse consumption is lowest for the Madras surveys where incomes are low (the average household income is Rs 771/− per annum, and the average *per capita* income is Rs 169/− per annum, table 5.14). Although data are only available for 12 villages, there is less variation between those villages than between villages of other areas. The average *per capita* income for the villages surveyed by the Visva Bharati AERCs is equally low; the value of cereal and pulse consumption is higher but the value of total food consumption as a percentage of total expenditure is also higher. These cover a mixture of poor (Bihar and Orissa), tribal and peri-urban, rich villages selling produce to Calcutta.

Table 5.13: Data on the Value of Food Consumption Extracted from Different AERC Studies

		Delhi	Madhya Pradesh	Sardar Patel	Uttar Pradesh	Madras	Visva Bharati
Total value of cereals and pulses consumed per household	Mean	891	462	487	880	349	560
	SD	2.3	1.3	1.2	2.5	0.5	1.9
	Coef. Var.	26	27.2	24.2	28.9	14.9	33
	n	28	13	13	14	12	18
The total value of cereal and pulse consumption as a percentage of the total value of food consumption	Mean	30.6	48.7	34.6	33.7	41.5	59
	SD	10.8	7.5	7.6	10.3	6.3	7.8
	Coef. Var.	35.3	15.4	21.9	30.5	15.2	13.3
	n	40	7	14	18	12	20
The value of total food consumption as a percentage of total expenditure	Mean	55.3	67.3	66.4	56.3	62.4	77.9
	SD	10.2	6.7	6.4	8.5	6.9	6.4
	Coef. Var.	18.5	10	9.6	15	11	8.2
	n	40	11	17	18	15	22
The value of superior cereal consumption as a percentage of the total value of food consumption	Mean	—	27.9	9.9	—	29.1	50.9
	SD	—	22	6.2	—	10	12.3
	Coef. Var.	—	78.8	62.9	—	34.4	24.1
	n	—	5	11	—	12	11
The value of inferior cereal consumption as a percentage of the total value of food consumption	Mean	—	17	19.8	—	9.5	4.7
	SD	—	12.4	10.3	—	8.5	5
	Coef. Var.	—	72.8	52	—	88.9	106.3
	n	—	5	11	—	12	11

In the AERC surveys, rice and wheat were classified as superior cereals and millets as inferior. Using this classification, we found that the value of superior cereal consumption as a percentage of the total value of food consumption is highest for villages surveyed by the Visva Bharati AERC because these are located in rice growing areas; the value of inferior cereal consumption is relatively low. The converse is true for Sardar Patel where the value of inferior cereal consumption as a percentage of the total value of food consumption is higher. Many of these villages are located in semi-desert regions where millets and barley are a predominant part of the diet. Villages surveyed by the Madhya Pradesh AERC are located in both arid and forest regions and the value of superior and inferior cereal consumption is less divergent.

These data on the value of food consumption were correlated with other socio-economic data for the same villages. Some of the results (table 5.15) are not new but are significant and substantiate other data. Household incomes are significantly and positively correlated with the total value of cereals and pulses consumed per household which indicates that as incomes rise the consumption of these foods increases. However, we cannot assume that higher income villages or higher income groups will automatically be better nourished than those less well off because it depends on how the additional income is spent.

With rising average and *per capita* incomes, other food items are consumed and the value of cereal and pulse consumption as a percentage of the total value of food consumption decreases (the relationships are significant but negative). As the percentage of families earning less than Rs 750/— per year increases per village, then the average absolute value of cereal and pulse consumption decreases (the relationship is negatively significant at the 1 per cent level) but as a percentage of the total value of food consumption it increases. As mean household and *per capita* incomes increase, then the value of superior cereal consumption as a percentage of the total value of food consumption decreases.

The villages surveyed by the Agro-Economic Research Centres were divided into south and north Indian villages, and in each area into cereal (wheat or millet) and rice villages either irrigated, or non-irrigated (see table 5.16). We found that the disparities in total household value of cereal and pulse consumption are wide and representative of income differences. The average household and *per capita* incomes are higher for the northern villages (which comprise villages from the Punjab and Haryana) as is the total value of cereal and pulse consumption. The value of total food consumption as a percentage of total expenditure is similar for both northern and southern villages although the value of cereal and pulse consumption as a percentage of the total value of food consumption is usually less for the northern villages. This indicates that

Table 5.14: Mean Income Data for Some of the Agro-Economic Research Centres

		Delhi	Madhya Pradesh	Sardar Patel	Uttar Pradesh	Madras	Visva Bharati
Average annual household income (Rupees)	Mean	—	—	1493.88	—	770.5	925.91
	SD	—	—	578.5	—	223.5	337
	Coef. Var.	—	—	38.7	—	29.01	36.4
	n	—	—	16	—	15	23
Average *per capita* income (Rupees)	Mean	—	—	269.6	—	169.2	168.9
	SD	—	—	1.052	—	0.62	0.462
	Coef. Var.	—	—	39.04	—	36.6	27.35
	n	—	—	16	—	15	23

Table 5.15: Correlation Analysis Between the Value of Food Consumption and Socio-Economic Variables Based on Data from 130 AERC Village Surveys

		Number Simple Households	Average Household Income per Annum	Percentage of Households Earning Less than Rs 750/- per Annum	Per Capita Income
Total value of cereals and pulses consumed per household	Correlation coefficient	-0.4765	0.7384	-0.5649	0.3239
	n	48	31	31	39
	Level of significance	0.1%	0.1%	1%	None
The total value of cereal and pulse consumption as a percentage of the total value of food consumption	Correlation coefficient	0.2477	-0.5946	0.4510	-0.6033
	n	51	28	28	40
	Level of significance	None	1%	2%	0.1%
The value of total food consumption as a percentage of total expenditure	Correlation coefficient	0.2081	0.0825	-0.1411	-0.2349
	n	59	36	36	50
	Level of significance	None	None	None	10%
The value of superior cereal consumption as a percentage of the total value of food consumption	Correlation coefficient	0.2245	-0.4781	0.4804	-0.5445
	n	23	25	25	31
	Level of significance	None	5%	None	1%
The value of inferior cereal consumption as a percentage of the total value of food consumption	Correlation coefficient	-0.2504	0.1203	-0.2273	0.1610
	n	23	25	25	31
	Level of significance	None	None	None	None

Table 5.16: The Value of Food Consumption for Different Types of Village Surveyed by the Agro-Economic Research Centres

		N	S	NCI	NCni	NRI	NRni	SCI	SCni	SRI	SRni
The total value of cereals and pulses consumed per household	Mean	665.8	349.2	748	609.9	782.5	573.9	—	354.8	359	—
	SD	2.52	0.52	2.04	2.6	3.16	1.82	—	0.51	0.47	—
	Coef. Var.	37.8	14.9	27.2	42.6	40.4	31.74	—	14.3	13.19	—
	n	62	12	15	22	11	14	—	5	6	—
The total value of cereal and pulse consumption as a percentage of the total value of food consumption	Mean	39.7	41.5	27.77	33.8	48.5	55.12	—	42.43	42.09	—
	SD	15.8	6.3	9.6	11.45	10.8	14.6	—	6.59	6.2	—
	Coef. Var.	39.9	15.2	34.6	33.9	22.2	26.5	—	15.53	14.7	—
	n	68	12	21	18	14	15	—	5	6	—
The value of total food consumption as percentage of total expenditure	Mean	63.95	62.4	54.68	61.3	68.97	74.78	—	60.93	63.9	—
	SD	13.2	6.9	7.67	13.7	10.22	11.31	—	4.8	9.4	—
	Coef. Var.	20.64	11.03	14.03	22.3	14.82	15.12	—	7.9	14.74	—
	n	72	15	22	19	14	17	—	5	7	—
The value of superior cereal consumption as a percentage of the total value of food consumption	Mean	35.3	29.13	—	7.81	39.78	47.18	—	23.02	35.6	—
	SD	22.9	10.02	—	6.6	8.04	19.39	—	11.11	4.6	—
	Coef. Var.	65	34.4	—	84.5	20.21	41.1	—	48.3	12.9	—
	n	18	12	—	5	2	10	—	5	6	—
The value of inferior cereal consumption as a percentage of the total value of food consumption	Mean	10.97	9.5	—	26.3	7.09	4.45	—	16.13	3.52	—
	SD	11.4	8.5	—	9.4	8.83	4.1	—	8.65	2.98	—
	Coef. Var.	104.3	88.9	—	35.6	124.5	92.2	—	53.6	84.7	—
	n	18	12	—	5	2	10	—	5	6	—

Key: N = North Indian Village   S = South Indian Village   C = Cereal
R = Rice   I = Irrigated   ni = Non-Irrigated

Table 5.17: Mean Income Data for Different Types of Village Surveyed by the Agro-Economic Research Centres

		N	S	NCI	NCni	NRI	NRni	SCI	SCni	SRI	SRni
Average household income	Mean	1085.9	770.47	796.7	1283.5	1080.6	957.3	—	919.2	689.6	—
	SD	444.8	223.5	69.6	537.74	351.6	366.2	—	275.5	193.4	—
	Coef. Var.	40.96	29.01	8.74	41.9	32.5	38.3	—	29.97	28.05	—
	n	41	15	3	15	7	16	—	5	7	—
Average *per capita* income	Mean	205.5	169.2	171.67	243.3	194	181.5	—	204.2	157	—
	SD	80.85	61.88	11.5	104.5	40.13	65.1	—	87.5	46.2	—
	Coef. Var.	39.3	36.6	6.7	42.97	20.69	35.9	—	42.8	29.42	—
	n	41	15	3	15	7	16	—	5	7	—

Key: N = North Indian Village.   S = South Indian Village   C = Cereal
R = Rice   I = Irrigated   ni = Non-Irrigated

the northern villages purchase more expensive foods although they spend only marginally more on superior cereals (wheat) than southern villages.

The value of cereal and pulse consumption is higher in irrigated than non-irrigated villages although incomes are not necessarily higher (these data are available for fewer villages). The average household income of north cereal non-irrigated villages is higher than the corresponding irrigated villages and the total value of cereal and pulse consumption is less. The value of total food consumption as a percentage of total expenditure is higher in the north cereal, non-irrigated villages than in the corresponding irrigated villages which indicates that other, more expensive food items are purchased.

Classification by Village Location and Accessibility

We attempted to classify African villages by degree of accessibility and location in the belief that isolated villages would have less access to marketing centres and therefore would sell fewer crops, purchase less food and in general be dependent on their own production. Villages of the opposite type, i.e. ones that are more accessible, should sell more crops, purchase more food and, in general, have diets different in quality and quantity to those of more isolated villages. This was demonstrated in a comparative study of 15 Tanzanian villages which showed that the sales of Shamba produce were heavily dependent on two factors: a regular market and the availability of road communications suitable for vehicles (Tanzania Central Statistical Bureau, 1963).

We divided these same villages into accessible and isolated (table 5.18) but although dietary differences were apparent, these were not significant. We also compared the diets of isolated and accessible villages from other parts of Africa (table 5.18). The isolated villages were distant from main roads and urban centres but still managed to market some crops through itinerant merchants. Larger amounts of cereals and vegetables were consumed in the isolated villages while the more accessible ones consumed more meat and fish.

Location relative to a main road was observed by Cros to be an important variable. He compared the diets of three villages at different distances from the main road (10 km, 3 km and 200 metres) and found that calorie and protein intakes were highest in the village nearest the main road although consumption of palm oil was greater in the more distant village. The two villages nearest the road were found to consume larger amounts of millet, legumes and condiments than in the village 10 km distant (Cros, 1967b). Of our sample of accessible villages, nine were located on a main road and six others were located at distances varying from 1 to 8 km from the road. Comparison of mean food consumption data shows that intakes of cereals, roots/tubers, legumes,

Table 5.18: Food Consumption (Grams per Caput per Day) in African Villages with Different Degrees of Accessibility

	n	Cereals	Roots/Tubers	Legumes	Vegetables	Meat	Fish
Tanzanian[a] villages with easy market access	6	3696	482	780	1638	48	212
Tanzanian villages with difficult market access	5	2874	628	277	1630	13	54
Isolated villages from other parts of Africa	6	2186	372	215	985	17	39
Accessible villages from other parts of Africa	17	1479	474	308	703	28	141
Accessible African villages situated on a main road	9	651	453	68	341 (n = 8)	13	176 (n = 4)
Accessible African villages not situated on a main road[b]	6	3160	475	718	1280	48	130 (n = 5)

Notes:
a These data were obtained from a comparative survey of 15 Tanzanian villages. (Tanzania Central Statistical Bureau, 1963.)
b These were still classified as accessible because they were situated near railroads, had easy access to markets or had good transport facilities.

Table 5.19: Correlation Analysis Between the Value of Food Consumption and Socio-Economic Variables Based on Data from 130 AERC Village Surveys

		Distance from Town	Distance from Main Road
Total value of cereals and pulses consumed per household	Correlation coefficient	−0.0727	0.2165
	n	83	84
	Level of significance	None	None
The total value of cereal and pulse consumption as a percentage of the total value of food consumption	Correlation coefficient	−0.0092	0.1682
	n	90	92
	Level of significance	None	None
The value of total food consumption as a percentage of total expenditure	Correlation coefficient	−0.0024	0.1378
	n	102	104
	Level of significance	None	None
The value of superior cereal consumption as a percentage of the total value of food consumption	Correlation coefficient	−0.3099	−0.0817
	n	38	39
	Level of significance	10%	None
The value of inferior cereal consumption as a percentage of the total value of food consumption	Correlation coefficient	0.4224	0.2592
	n	38	39
	Level of significance	1%	None

vegetables and meat were higher in the non-main road villages (see table 5.18) but differences were not significant.

We managed to classify 'main road' and 'isolated' villages in Latin America and found a great variety in types of cereals consumed in the main road villages. The mean *per capita* consumption of sugar in the isolated villages was found to be less (39 g *per capita* per day) than in 16 'main road' villages (64 g per person per day).

A further correlation was made between the value of total food consumption (including subsistence and purchased foods) with distance from a town and distance from a main road using data extracted from 130 AERC surveys. The results are not conclusive although the value of inferior cereal consumption (millets) was found to increase (as a percentage of the total value of food consumption) in villages further away from towns and was significantly correlated'at the 1 per cent level. Expectedly, the value of superior cereal consumption decreases (significant at 10 per cent).

Conclusions

In this chapter we attempted to produce a typology of village diets but paucity of socio-economic data prevented the isolation of key variables and our classification was by type of climate, main food staple, economy, value of food consumption, village location and accessibility.

Attempts to classify village diets by main food staple were significant and the differences between maize and potato diets were especially significant. Maize diets were found to be significantly different from rice and cassava diets and distinguishable by the level of niacin intake. Maize and cassava diets were found to be significantly different, with protein intakes and adequacies lower in the cassava diets and Vitamin C intakes and adequacies higher.

Classification of rural diets by type of economy was less conclusive although pure subsistence villages were found to be significantly better off than semi-subsistence or semi-cash crop villages. Although isolated villages, when compared with more accessible villages, were found to consume different quantities of food, village location and accessibility could not be proved to be the key variables. Other Malthusian or migration factors or raising man/land ratios faster in the more fortunately located villages may have been operational.

Data on the total value of food consumption were collected from a much larger number of studies but unfortunately could not be correlated with the nutritional adequacy of the diets. The value of cereal and pulse consumption was found to be greater in the high income villages and those with a small population earning less than Rs 750/— per annum. High income villages are therefore likely to consume more cereals and pulses. If increased consumption of these foods leads to a better diet — mainly in terms of calorie and protein consumption — then high income villages (north India) will be nutritionally better off than low income (southern Indian) villages. Similarly, one could expect irrigated villages to be nutritionally better off than non-irrigated villages since the data indicate that the value of cereal and pulse consumption is higher in the irrigated villages. With better, more reliable data of different types including ultimate as well as proximate data from a random sample of villages, different and more reliable typologies of village diets could be identified.

6 INTRA-VILLAGE IDENTIFICATION OF NUTRITION PROBLEMS

A comparative evaluation of data from nutrition surveys in the less developed world has provided us with certain insights into village nutrition problems. We have so far concentrated on differences between villages and the identification of nutrition problems by village type. Once these have been identified, we have to find out whether some groups are more vulnerable than others, and if so, why, so that planners can best time, locate and implement different programmes. We must be able to answer two sets of questions: firstly, why does one family suffer more malnutrition than another and can those at-risk families be quickly, cheaply and reliably identified? Secondly, within a family, why are certain members more malnourished than others? Planners also need to identify the factors that are responsible for differences in food/nutrient consumption between seasons, between households and between members of the same household and show how their combined effect influences some households and individuals more than others. Therefore in this chapter we attempt to identify (1) actual nutritional differences within a village in terms of variation between households, differences within households, and seasonal variations and (2) the factors responsible for these differences.

Actual Nutritional Differences Within a Village

Inter-Household Differences

Study of dietary differences between families in one village will suggest not only what types of improvement programmes are needed and where these should be implemented but will also indicate their directional effects. For example with income increments, poorer sections of a village population may well switch to diets of a type already consumed by the better-off sectors of the village which may mean, not more and better food, but more packaging, polished rice and bottle-feeding. Time-series data would provide better information (Ojha, 1969) but these are comparatively rare so that data on inter-household differences must suffice. These are generally poor as samples are often as small as five households (Lawson, 1957). Although striking differences between them were observed, these could not be extrapolated for the whole village. Other surveys indicate the range of dietary adequacies within the village (the percentage fulfilment of calorie requirements ranged from 62 to 162 per cent for one Guatemalan village — Flores, 1957)

Table 6.1: Mean Percentage Distribution of Households in Eight Rural Areas of Iran[a] According to their Calorie Intakes

Number of Villages by Area[b]	Calories				
	Below 1500	1500—2000	2001—2500	2501—3000	3001+
12	1.4	8.3	26.4	25	38.9
7	2.1	25.5	31.9	19.1	21.2
6	0	15	32.5	22.5	30
8	12.9	27.1	20	21.3	18.7
12	6.9	30.5	25	16.7	20.8
12	27.1		24.2	28.3	20.6
8	20		30	31	19
3	29.2		26.4	27.4	17

Notes:

[a] The data were obtained from seven nutrition surveys conducted by the Food and Nutrition Institute of Teheran in conjunction with the FAO. These data were obtained from Reports to the Government of Iran Nos. 4, 5, 7, 8, 9, 10 and 11.

[b] One of these surveys provided data for two areas.

while more accurate surveys (Burgess and Wheeler, 1970) include the standard deviation or coefficient of variation for this range. Other surveys with information on inter-household differences in nutrition include those by White (1954), studies by Gunasekera (1958) who surveyed six villages in Ceylon and studies in Peru by Collazos (1953). Several village surveys provide data on the percentage distribution of households according to their nutrient intake and the percentage adequacy of nutrient consumption. The Food and Nutrition Institute of Iran, sometimes in conjunction with the FAO, systematically provide those data for a series of surveys. Data from seven of these provides information for eight areas of Iran. Although these are aggregated and we have only extracted information on calorie intakes, they indicate the range of household distribution by calorie intake within an area/village. Table 6.1 shows that, in general, a relatively high proportion of households in each area are consuming less than 2,000 calories per day.

It is obviously very difficult to assess the range of nutrient adequacies let alone attach socio-economic characteristics to this range. Some surveys compare the diets of different socio-economic groups within the village. Those conducted by the Instituto Nacional de Nutricion de Colombia frequently and consistently present survey data in this way, but unfortunately the samples are too small to provide results which are statistically representative of each group.

Socio-economic status is difficult to measure especially when incomes are varied, employment is irregular and family structure changes frequently (Desai, 1970). In general, families of low socio-economic status may be landless, illiterate, of low caste or of small *per capita* income. They have fewer resources to divert to the special needs of children even if these needs are recognised which is less likely since access to information is also low in such groups.

Intra-Household Differences

Differences in nutritional status between members of the same family occur at times of food surplus and deficit. If similar individuals (i.e. of the same age, sex, status, etc.) of families of similar types (same structure, size, income group, etc.) are found to be nutritionally at risk then we can identify vulnerable groups upon which attention can be focused and action directed. Those commonly identified for planners include pre-school children and pregnant or lactating mothers. These efforts at identification make no attempt to evaluate the factors responsible for causing some groups to be more malnourished than others. It is constantly assumed that it is lack of food rather than the unequal distribution of both time and resources which is the constraint. These factors will be discussed later; here we will examine (1) the evidence for differences in nutritional status between family members and (2) the proximate (nutritional) causes of these.

Differences in Nutritional Status

Anthropometric data are a good measure of nutritional status especially height/weight data which occur frequently in the village studies. It is these data which were used to evaluate differences in nutritional status between members of the same family. Achieved height and weight measurements were expressed as a percentage of the expected measures for different age groups and will be referred to as weight/age or height/age. For older family members, achieved weights were expressed as a percentage of expected weights for their heights and will be referred to as weight/height (for the reference tables, see Jelliffe, 1966).

Data for our analysis were obtained from a small sample of Latin American and African villages. Where possible data were extracted by age group (0–4 years, 4–6, 7–9, 10–14 and 15–19 years) and sex since general findings from several surveys in Haiti by Ballweg (1972) and in Gambia by McGregor (1968) indicated that pre-school girls were more likely to suffer weight loss than boys of the same age who may also be as much as 1.3 cm taller. Analysis of data from 94 Latin American villages showed that females aged 0–4 years fulfilled 87 per cent of their expected weight/age measurements compared with the 90 per cent level achieved by boys of the same age. The differences (measured by the t-paired test) were found to be significant at the 0.5 per cent level. Differences in achieved height/age and weight/height measurements between males and females were not found to be significant for the pre-school children or any other age group from 5 to 19 years in the Latin American sample. In the African sample, differences in weight/age and height/age measurements between boys and girls were not significant in the pre-school age group. Differences in weight/height measurements were found to be significant (at the 2 per cent level) in the 10—14 age group only, but the sample was extremely small. Here males achieved 102 per cent of their expected weight/height measurements and females achieved 96 per cent.

As with pre-school children, other evidence (Marsden, 1965) suggested that adult females are consistently lighter in terms of weight/height than men. This was corroborated by Masseyeff in the Cameroons, who found that men have a 'mean deficit of 5.7 per cent from expected weight for height while women have a deficit of 10.7 per cent' (1959, p. 52). We were led to expect such differences from village data which indicate that both foods and nutrients are preferentially distributed to males rather than females. However, our analysis of the village data on nutritional status does not uniformly support this. Height/weight data for both adult males and non-pregnant females are available in 26 African village surveys. Analysis of these data unexpectedly indicated that the mean percentage height/weight figures achieved by adult females (94 per cent) are 5 per cent higher than those achieved by adult males (89 per cent) and this difference was found in the t-paired test to be significant at the 0.5 per cent level. These differences are more significant (at the 2.5 per cent level) in the 30—39 year age group when males achieved 83 per cent of their expected weight/height measurement and females 92 per cent, than in the 20—29, 50—59 (significant at the 10 per cent level) or 40—49 year age groups (no significant differences). Similar results were obtained in an analysis of data from 31 Latin American villages: adult males met only 93 per cent of the expected height/weight measurements while adult females achieved 101 per cent. These differences were significant only at the 0.1 per cent level but differences were only significant for age groups aged 30—39 years and 50—59 years at the 1 and 5 per cent levels respectively.

These results are not what we would expect but they are based on an extremely small and non-random sample of village data. There may also be other explanations. Firstly, adult nutritional status does not always indicate present levels of consumption since height retardations may have occurred during childhood. Present weights assessed against retarded heights rather than expected weights for age may not present a reliable picture of present nutritional status. Secondly, if it is proteins rather than calories which are distributed to adult males rather than females, this will not be reflected in weight/height differences until severe muscle wasting contributes to weight loss. Thirdly, these anthropometric measures do not usually take seasonal weight loss into account. As this can be abrupt and dramatic, and perhaps worse for females rather than males, these data are certainly not very reliable. An alternative indicator is to measure the differences in nutrient consumption levels.

Differences in Nutrient Consumption

Household members require different quantities of foods and nutrients depending on their age, sex, physical and physiological status. These can be compared by expressing the nutrient requirements of each member as a fraction of the requirements of the adult male. For each member and household we can thus obtain a standardised consumption or Lusk coefficient (Gopalan, 1971). For a family of five members (adult male sedentary worker, adult female heavy worker, one adolescent and two children under five years of age) the consumption coefficient is $1+1.2+1+0.4+0.4 = 4$. In theory, any nutrient supply available to this family should be distributed in the ratio of $1:1.2:1.0:0.4:0.4$ but in practice this is not always the case since there are numerous factors operating to constrain the distribution of foods/nutrients in relation to requirements.

Quantitative data from village nutrition surveys on the intra-family distribution of either foods or nutrients are limited and of poor quality. A few surveys provide data on mean food/nutrient distribution between age/sex groups for a representative sample of the village population. These include surveys conducted in Puerto Rico by Fernandez (1965, 1966 and 1968), one village survey in Nicaragua by Nietschmann (1972) and one African survey in Nigeria by the University of Ibadan (1968). Studies providing data on intra-household food and/or nutrient consumption between individuals are also few in number and generally omit data for persons whose food consumption is difficult to measure (breast feeding infants) or whose nutritional status is less important relative to the more vulnerable groups because they are not members of the work-force or soon to die (people over the age of 50 years). Surveys providing data on intra-household distribution include: an Indian village survey by Devadas and others (1969) surveys in Oceania by Reid (1969) and Bailey (1963), and African studies by Nicol (1959) and the University of Ibadan (1963). Other useful non-village surveys with information on the intra-family distribution of food/nutrients include: a study in Nigeria by Nicol (1956), a study in New Guinea by Hitchcock and Oram (1967), one in India by Belavady

(1959) and several in the Philippines by Bailey (1966) Bulatao-Jayme and others (1966 and 1968).

Qualitative data are more common and suggest that men, even allowing for their higher energy requirements receive an unfair share of the total family food. This may not be unfair if adult males are the only wage earners. If this is the case it makes more economic sense to feed the workers at the expense of their dependants who would receive even less if the adult males did no work at all through sheer lack of energy. Pregnant and lactating females and pre-school children are stated to be the worst off (University of Ibadan, 1968, p. 91). Analysis of data from a non-random sample of African villages indicates that in relation to their requirements, adults (excluding pregnant and lactating females) consume more than any other age group. Unfortunately data were too few to test the statistical significance of this.

We can express the calorie intakes and requirements of one age group as a percentage of the intakes and requirements of the adult male and calculate the difference by the formula

$$\left(\frac{\text{calorie intakes of pre-school children}}{\text{calorie intakes of adult males}} \times 100 \right) -$$

$$\left(\frac{\text{calorie requirements of pre-school children}}{\text{calorie requirements of adult males}} \times 100 \right)$$

$$= \text{Difference (plus or minus)}$$

In theory, the amount of calories consumed by the pre-school child as a proportion of adult calorie intake should be the same as the figure for pre-school requirements as a proportion of adult male requirements. If the difference is positive, then pre-school children are better off than adult males, but if the difference is negative, then the reverse is true. In this case ($n = 6$), we find that the mean difference for children aged 10–12 years is minus 18.3 per cent and for children aged 7–9 years is minus 15.7 per cent. Generally, calories are distributed in favour of adult females rather than children and in favour of older (10–12 years) rather than younger children (4–6 or 7–9 years): in only one village did we find that children aged 4–9 years were consuming more calories (in relation to their different requirements) than children aged 10–12 years.

The significance of the deviation from the expected nutrient distribution curve (where available nutrients are equally distributed in relation to the requirement ratio) can be measured by Skewness and Kurtosis tests. These were conducted on detailed data (percentage fulfilment of the requirements of nine nutrients) for 12 age/sex groups from three studies. The results (table 6.2) indicate that the distribution

Table 6.2: Skewness and Kurtosis Tests to Examine the Distribution of Nutrients in Three Latin American Villages

Village No.		Calories	Protein	Calcium	Iron	Vitamin A	Thiamine	Riboflavine *	Niacin	Vitamin C
1	Coefficient of skewness	-0.19813	—	0.0547	-0.13819	2.2888	-0.12474	2.01709	-0.50494	0.72336
	Level of significance	0.05	—	0.05	0.05	0.05	0.05	0.05	0.05	0.05
	Coefficient of Kurtosis	-0.60007	—	-1.17722	0.15265	5.95545	0.53438	4.38693	-0.02322	-0.3016
	Level of significance	0.05	—	0.05	0.05	0.05	0.05	0.05	0.05	0.05
2	Coefficient of skewness	1.84004	0.17310	0.41178	0.17449	2.47923	-0.89734	0.91801	-1.40804	0.68527
	Level of significance	0.05	0.05	0.05	0.05	0.05	0.05	0.05	0.05	0.05
	Coefficient of Kurtosis	2.42083	-0.98642	-0.13255	-1.23859	5.97226	0.53027	0.62962	2.78408	0.89751
	Level of significance	0.05	0.05	0.05	0.05	0.05	0.05	0.05	0.05	0.05
3	Coefficient of skewness	-1.35018	1.15063	0.60421	1.3128	1.44787	0.05377	2.18409	-0.85926	0.19164
	Level of significance	0.05	0.05	0.05	0.05	0.05	0.05	0.05	0.05	0.05
	Coefficient of Kurtosis	2.84301	0.76826	-0.91462	3.23253	2.00404	-0.24769	5.34282	1.84537	-0.56826
	Level of significance	0.05	0.05	0.05	0.05	0.05	0.05	0.05	0.05	0.05

was significantly skewed at the 5 per cent level. Although the direction of skewness was undetermined, it was concluded in the studies that pre-school children and pregnant or lactating females are the worst sufferers.

Analysis of data from 11 African villages showed that adult males fulfilled calorie and protein requirements at 101 and 251 per cent respectively, while adult females achieved lower levels of 96 and 136 per cent. Differences between male and female calorie and protein fulfilment levels were not found to be significant. In other geographical areas, similar data were available for only one Indian village survey (Rao and Rao, 1958) and for four Latin American surveys (Fernandez, 1965, 1966 and 1968 and Nietschmann, 1972). The survey of Pennathur village in Tamil Nadu State in India showed that adult males fulfilled their requirements of all nutrients at a higher level than adult females while in the three Puerto Rican villages surveyed by Fernandez, adult males aged 20–39 and 40–59 years achieved higher levels of calorie and protein adequacy than females of the corresponding ages.

The mean calorie intakes per caput indicate the availability of calories per individual if these were equally distributed. However, in 19 Latin American villages, pre-school calorie intakes expressed as a percentage of per caput intakes show that they are consuming only 46 per cent of the calories theoretically available to them. For seven African villages this figure is 62 per cent. Twenty-nine studies from Latin America and 10 from Africa provide data on the percentage fulfilment of nutrient requirements in the pre-school age group. For the Latin American villages, calorie, protein, calcium, iron and thiamine requirements of pre-school children were fulfilled at 80, 84, 70, 135 and 105 per cent respectively. These figures were lower than the *per capita* fulfilment levels which were 90, 99, 110, 158 and 144 per cent respectively and the differences as measured by the t-paired test were found to be significant between 1 and 0.1 per cent. Differences in fulfilment of calorie requirements in the pre-school age group and the mean *per capita* figure were found to be significant at the 0.1 per cent level in a sample of 10 African villages.

We emphasise the importance of intra-household nutrient distribution by estimating the impact of redistributing the nutrient supply available to each village in relation to the requirement ratio. To do this, it was essential to have data on the intakes and requirements of the pre-school sector. It was impossible to obtain data on the 0–4 year old pre-school population because it would have been difficult to measure the nutrient contribution from breast milk. To avoid this problem we used data for the 4–6 year 'pre-school' age group. We also needed to know the number of pre-school children in the survey and the number of people in the *per capita* sample. All these data were available for only six African and one Latin American village. In each of the African villages, the pre-school age group fulfilled 87, 74, 96, 68, 76 and 78 per cent of their calorie requirements. In comparison, the mean fulfilment levels for the rest of the population in each village were 128, 87, 108, 111, 94 and 87 per cent respectively. If we redistribute the total calorie supply available to the village such that all sectors of the population fulfil their different requirements for calories to the same extent, then the following *per capita* levels are achieved: 125, 78, 107, 108, 93 and 86 per cent respectively. To achieve these figures, the village population excluding the pre-school age group have reduced their calorie intakes in each village by −3, −9, −1, −3, −1 and −1 per cent only which has boosted the fulfilment levels of the pre-school age group in each village by 38, 4, 11, 40, 17 and 8 per cent respectively. The mean reduction in the percentage fulfilment of calorie requirements for the remainder of the population is only 3 per cent from 102 to 99 per cent while the percentage level of fulfilment in the 4–6 year age group has increased by 20 per cent from 79 to 99 per cent.

Seasonal Differences

We have already shown in chapter 5 that seasonal differences in nutrient adequacy are more significant in mono-cropping, rain dependent villages with a unimodal rainfall than continuous cropping villages with a bimodal distribution of rain. Here we shall look at individual examples (see Appendix A, pp. 133–47) and relate problems of seasonal food supply more closely with the pattern of life in the village.

Tables A1–A3 provide examples of differences in calorie adequacy in villages with a unimodal distribution of rain. For example, in the Senegalese villages (table A2), only one millet crop is harvested each year, and there is a distinct shortage of this cereal and other foods during the wet season, before new supplies of millet are ready and at the time of heavy farm work. Most of these studies (especially A3) demonstrate how supplies of certain nutrients vary with the seasonal availability and harvesting of certain foodstuffs. In the south Indian village (table A3), calorie intakes are highest in the first season at the time of the rice harvest; protein intakes are high in the first and fourth seasons since paddy and pulses are harvested then and available at moderate cost; calcium levels peak in the second and third seasons when ragi is cultivated; Vitamin A intakes are high in the last two seasons when green leafy vegetables are abundant; niacin consumption is high when rice and groundnuts are harvested and riboflavin when cholam and groundnuts are picked.

In contrast to these 'unimodal rainfall villages' is the southern Cameroon village, Bokindja (table A5), which has a bimodal distribution of rain. Seasonal variations in food/nutrient consumption still occur but calorie supplies are more regular because two wet seasons make two crop cycles feasible (two maize and groundnut harvests) and because the diet is mixed and based on both cereals and roots/ tubers which are substituted for each other when either is in short supply. Bokindja (table A5) is, however, a fairly traditional agricultural village with fishing and hunting as secondary occupations. In comparison, Tikondi (table A6) another south Cameroon village also subject to a bimodal rainy season, is less traditional and cultivates cash crops of cocoa, coffee and tobacco. Here protein intakes are highest just after the tobacco harvest since money is available to purchase beef. Protein supplies vary more by season since there is less time for the traditional occupations of hunting and fishing. Supplies of other nutrients are also highly seasonal and there is a definite shortage of food at the end of the second wet season (September and October) before the second maize harvest.

Factors Responsible for Nutritional Differences Within a Village

Socio-Economic and Family Factors Affecting Inter-Household Differences

Our data indicate that within any village, inter- and intra-household differences in nutritional status occur as a result of different levels of nutrient consumption the causes of which we have yet to understand. Some village studies compare the diets of different socio-economic groups, as characterised by differences in incomes, occupation and religion but we would like to identify nutritionally at-risk families by other 'family' variables such as size, structure and age of mother, etc. Substantive evidence is limited and concentrated on families at-risk of rearing malnourished and especially pre-school children. Nutritional risk affecting other members of these families has not been investigated and it may be for example that certain factors characteristic of families with malnourished infants are not definitive of those with malnourished adolescents. Whatever the characteristics of those families, they are generally the ones least likely to approach socially neutral services for child nutrition so their quick and easy identification will facilitate the distribution of curative and preventative treatment.

Poverty stricken families, those of low income, low caste, landless and perhaps only seasonally employed for low wages are nutritionally worse off in comparison with the wealthier, land-owning and salaried households. Morley (1968) found that in a Nigerian village more children with standard weight for age measurements came from successful farming families who owned more land, were owner operators and had a surfeit of food while Hedayat (1971) found that in Iran, correlations between economic status and birth weight were significant and positive. Although such studies are few, they have important policy implications. Wray (1969) found significant correlations between the incidence of protein calorie malnutrition in Columbian pre-school children and income, food expenditure levels and the percentage of income spent on food, whilst Wray and Aguirre found that an increase of 8 US cents per day per person made a remarkable improvement to the diet (1969).

Custom and income can affect diet independently, as when a poor Indian caste attempts to gain social status by adopting vegetarian habits usually associated with richer groups. Wealthier families may not enjoy significantly better diets in remote or monocultural villages, with limited access to new foods or new sources of income. Freedman writes of Indonesia that 'the few better-off households seemed to maintain an ordinary diet not strikingly different from that of the great majority of households. ... Food habits, like other trends of social behaviour, may be so standardised in a particular milieu that differences in economic resources fail to affect them materially' (195(5), p. 17). Amounts of foods rather than types of foods consumed will vary with income although there is a tendency to consume more superior cereals as incomes rise. For example, Yeshwanth evaluated the cereal consumption levels per adult unit for nine different income groups in an Indian village from Rs 250 to more than Rs 5,000. Between Rs 250 and Rs 1,000, cereal consumption did not show much variation. Above Rs 2,000, levels of cereal intake were markedly higher. Similarly, the percentage of superior cereals in the diet was found to increase at higher income levels. A comparative survey of Ceylonese villages by Gunasakera (1958) showed that as income rises, the quantity of food eaten increases but there is no change in the diet pattern. The adequacy of calorie intake was found to rise with *per capita* daily income. At just over one rupee *per capita* per day the calorie intake of the family is nearly adequate and remains so at higher income levels.

Surveys of this type are common (see also Usha, 1964; Singh, 1971) but longitudinal data are best: see the study of Govindapur village by Ojha (1969) where baseline data collected in 1959 are compared with 1966 resurvey data. The results showed a tendency towards increased cereal consumption with increasing income levels; daily intakes of pulses and flesh foods were found to have increased in the higher income ranges but had decreased in lower income groups. These data are good but what we need to determine is the income-level cut-off point at which families purchase superior cereals or protein-rich foods or spend any additional income increments on items other than food. Investigation of consumer behaviour could indicate the necessity for improving purchasing patterns rather than raising the purchasing potential of some income groups.

Differences in food consumption between occupational groups are bound to reflect differences in income levels but may also be governed by type of work. Flores (1962) compared the diets of railway workers, agriculturalists and other occupational groups in a Guatemalan village and found minimal differences in calorie and/or protein intakes whereas in a Tamil Nadu village, Yeshwanth and Rajagopalan (1964) found a wide variation in consumption of cereals between manual labourers and other occupational groups. Labourers were found to consume 27.88 oz. of cereals per day compared with 21.34 for those employed in arts and crafts and 17.2 for service workers. The latter two groups consumed a higher proportion of superior cereals (rice) than did the labourers for whom millet was the main staple. In the Congo, it was found that significant differences between agriculturalists and salaried workers were related to the quality and quantity of animal products in the diet (Ministère de la Cooperation, 1967, p. 203).

One would expect the landowners and owner-operators to be nutritionally better off than those they employ since they control the means of production and have direct access to the product. Thus in one Indian village (Applied Nutrition Institute, 1966–67), the landowners had higher nutrient intake levels than the landless labourers due to their larger intakes of cereals, pulses, milk, flesh foods, sugar and oils. Similarly, Huenemann compares the diets of six Bolivian households of farm-workers with two households of farm owners and concluded that except for calcium, riboflavin and Vitamin C, 'the average intake of farm owners' households almost met or exceeded the recommended allowances. Farm-workers' diets, on the other hand, were low in all nutrients except vitamin C' (1957, p. 27). In general, price rises over a 7 year period were profitable for landowners selling their marketable surplus at higher prices but were nutritionally detrimental for their employees whose cash wage increments did not absorb the increased food prices or whose wages in kind were not increased to provide the extra food they could not otherwise afford (Ojha, 1969).

Even in different religious groups income may be the factor determining dietary differences. Singh provides data on food and nutrient intakes for 15 religious/caste groups in an Indian village. These were regrouped into scheduled castes, Moslems and non-scheduled castes. The Moslems were found to consume more cereals, more wheat, more meat and twice as much milk/milk products as the other two groups but these differences were consistent with the purchasing power rather than the food habits of each group. Another survey by Collis (1962) compared Moslem and non-Moslem diets in a Nigerian village; the results show that non-Moslems consume large amounts of cereal based beer; that Moslems consume larger quantities of meat and cow's milk (an expensive way to get proteins and calories), but they do not examine possible economic reasons for these differences. In general, however, religious restrictions can prohibit the consumption of certain foods and therefore of certain nutrients throughout the year or during feasts such as Ramadan. Stringently observed, rules can have more detrimental effects for some age groups (e.g. children), than on others such as overweight people in higher income groups.

Other factors affecting nutritional risk families are often income-linked. For example, low-income households may have to send mothers out to work. Several surveys correlate type and extent of maternal employment with children's nutritional status. Wray and Aguirre (1969) found in Candelaria, a small town in Colombia, that 44 per cent of children whose mothers worked were malnourished: 52 per cent of the children whose mothers worked part-time were malnourished compared with 32 per cent of children whose mothers worked full-time. The authors conclude that 'mothers who must work full-time manage somehow to make adequate arrangements for the care of their children' (1969, p. 88) but to us the results suggest that (a) those households with working mothers are poorer than those with non-working mothers simply because they have to go out to work and that (b) those households with mothers who can only work part-time may have lower incomes than those whose mothers work full-time.

Large family size aggravates almost all other factors affecting nutrition. The more children in the family, the lower the *per capita* food intakes (Fellowship Course in Food Science and Applied Nutrition, 1966, p. 88) since the amount of disposable income and volume of available food decreases with each additional family member. Rao and Gopalan (1971) studied the calorie and protein content of the diets of 500 Indian families from one socio-economic group whose family income was below Rs 250/— month. They found that 'families with three or less children were observed to have better intakes of calories and proteins than families with four or more children. The difference in calorie intake per adult unit between families with three or less children and those with four or more children was nearly 300. The difference in protein intake was of the order of 10 g daily. In most families, differences of this order implied a difference between deficiency and adequacy. These results show that limitation of family size to three or less children would have enabled practically all the families surveyed to afford an adequate dietary allowance and within their current economic means' (1971, pp. 342—3).

In such families, it is usually the new members who suffer most. Therefore it is not only total family size but the total number of children — especially the number of under five's — which is important. Burgess and Wheeler found that in one Malawi village, 'there is a tendency for families with a large number of children relative to the number of adults to be "calorie deficient" ' (1970, p. 69) and Wray (1969) discovered in Colombia that if mothers were able to limit their family size, the nutritional status of pre-school children would improve. But the problem is circular: the higher the infant mortality rate, the higher will be the birth-rate as the family tries to increase its chances of at least one son surviving. The number of children under five is a crucial variable. If members of this already vulnerable group have to compete within the family, for scarce food, care and attention, their vulnerability will increase as family size increases. Thus Antrobus (1971) found that 'children who lived in homes where there was a total of not more than two children under 5 years of age, were consistently heavier up to 2 years of age than those who belonged to homes with more than two under-fives' (1971).

The youngest being least able to fend for themselves may suffer most and therefore birth order, where a higher birth order implies the presence of an already large number of children, is an important measure of vulnerability within any family's pre-school age group. Morley (1968) argues that in Nigeria, family size is not important unless a child is born above a birth order of seven. This is exceptionally high: Rao and Gopalan (1971) investigated 872 hospitalised cases of severe protein-calorie malnutrition in India and found that 39 per cent of the children belonged to birth orders three or below while 61 per cent belonged to birth orders four or above. Although data from a non-hospitalised control group were not analysed, the authors concluded that limitation of family size to three or fewer children could reduce the incidence of kwashiorkor by at least 60 per cent.

In theory, long birth intervals between children will reduce strain on the mother and competition between siblings for her attention and care. In general, short birth intervals will indicate at-risk families liable to produce at-risk infants and vulnerable mothers. If pregnancy stops mothers from breast-feeding (breast-feeding while pregnant is commonly believed to harm both foetus and infant) then infants born at short birth intervals are at-risk from insufficient breast-milk. Fifteen-month birth intervals are indicative of early weaning at 6 months of age in comparison with long intervals of 34 months which are indicative of at least 25 months of breast feeding. With short birth intervals, children aged 6 months of age are likely to be in competition with older siblings at 21 months of age. Until a further pregnancy terminates the breast-feeding of the 6 month child, the latter could also suffer breast-milk deprivation if the mother uses the breast as a comforter or food source for the 21 month infant. In some circumstances, increasing the birth interval and reducing family size by contraception campaigns may be the most nutritionally efficient use of resources.

Children of higher birth orders not only suffer competition from other siblings but are born to older mothers who have been subject to longer periods of nutritional deprivation, child-bearing and over-work. Those mothers may be less fit in terms of nutritional/health status to cope with the additional energy demands of child feeding and care and their milk production may be reduced. In one Colombian village, Wray compared the nutritional status of children whose mothers were below and above the age of 35 and found that 38.4 per cent of the former were malnourished compared with 51 per cent of the latter. This difference was strongly significant but was not corroborated by Burgess (1970) in Malawi. Hedayat (1971) on the other hand found that, in Iran, maternal age of 30 years was the turning point up to which a significant, systematically increasing trend in the birth weight was observed. Since a mother's nutritional status may determine her capacity for breast-feeding or child care, her condition on its own may be a useful indicator of the family's potential for producing at-risk children. Indeed it has been shown (Morley, 1968) that the group of mothers with substandard weight/height measurements three months after delivery had substandard weight infants. Morley also found similar patterns of low birth weight/poor weight gain in siblings. Families may also be at-risk where mothers are not educated and less able to understand the health and nutritional needs of children. Although the analysis was based on a small sample, Burgess (1970) found significantly less protein-calorie malnutrition in the group of Malawi children whose mothers had received some education. Few village mothers have the opportunity to attend school long enough to become literate but, especially in culturally stable environments that permit 'natural learning', failures to use culturally acceptable foods are usually due to fuel or labour shortages or low income rather than ignorance. Hedayat (1971) in Iran and Wray (1969) in Colombia, found that a mother's literacy was statistically more important than her level of education in decreasing the probability of malnutrition in her children. They did not indicate whether or not literate mothers were economically better off than illiterate ones.

The quality and quantity of child care and the nutritional status of the mother may depend not only on her age or education but on the availability of other female time and help to cope with agricultural labour demands or to look after the children. Polygamous and extended families may have a surfeit of adult and responsible females to provide continuous and adequate child care independent of seasonal agricultural demands on female labour and time. Conditions for resource allocation may be more flexible here than in the monogamous and nuclear family where additional female family labour, even though only temporarily required, is unavailable. Although those families are larger and have more mouths to feed, Hauck (1958) observed in a Siamese village,

Morley (1968) in his study of a Nigerian village, and Burgess (1970) in Malawi, that the incidence of protein calorie malnutrition is not related to the number of wives in the family. Such families can econ-omise on child care, food preparation, water carrying and fuel collecting. Polygamy is detrimental, however, if the husband is living elsewhere and the wife has to support her family on a poor plot of land (Bennett, 1968). Certainly campaigns for or against polygamy − or the extended family − should consider economic effects, including the real cost of child care.

In Haiti, Ballweg found that 'severe malnutrition was far more characteristic of the one parent than the two parent family' (1972, p. 238). Mothers are overworked in attempting to support and care for their dependants so that children may be deprived both of food and of other important forms of care. Therefore families of widows, divorcees or wives separated from their husbands are nutritionally at risk. Desai found the same situation in Jamaica where 'children living with neither parent grew better than those living with single mothers, but children living with both parents grew better than either of these groups' (1970, p. 141). In Nigeria, Morley compared two groups of children: the weights of children in group A fell below the tenth percentile on one or more occasions at 6, 9 or 12 months of age while group B children consisted of those whose weights at 6 months were between the fiftieth and seventy-fifth percentile or were above this upper limit. He found that in group A there were a larger number of mothers who were widowed or separated from their husbands and received no support. Grass widows whose migrant husbands fail to send back remittances are often as badly off as real widows in terms of economic support. One of the problems is that migration of the male sector causes a labour shortage and the women are left to get on with the farming (McCrae, 1966). If the women cannot cope alone, pro-duction will fall and food be in short supply. Women overworked in the agricultural sector will have less time for child care, cooking, cleaning, etc. and the nutritional situation will deteriorate.

Factors Affecting Intra-Household Differences

An adequate food supply caused, amongst other things by low incomes and poor food production levels, is the primary cause of malnutrition in some households especially large, poverty stricken families. However, we are looking for factors other than total food supply which (a) affect the quantity and quality of foods consumed by individual family members, and (b) cause intra-family differences in health status. Mal-distribution of foods/nutrients is an especially important factor since minor differences in the diet may make all the difference between malnutrition and health on a basically inadequate diet (McCrae, 1966).

Even marginally inadequate diets, if fairly distributed between family members, could perhaps prevent the appearance of the more serious cases of malnutrition.

In small scale societies, rules of behaviour are usually strict and formalise ways in which different categories of people should behave towards each other. The position of a husband *vis-à-vis* his wife or children is fixed and food is often distributed according to existing status definitions. A food consumer will thus receive food deemed worthy of his status or may receive larger amounts of food in comparison with everyone else. The senior male members of the household are frequently given the best diet in terms of both quality and quantity and boys often have priority over girls. Status foods include meat which at most meals is distributed first to those of higher status (household head or guest). In cases where small children cannot anyway consume meat or when the amounts available would if equally distributed make only a small contribution to the nutrient supply, this differential distribution is less crucial.

The 'how, when and where' of food allocation affects the amounts and types consumed by different family members. The number and timing of meals, methods of serving, number of guests, rules of hospitality, etc. all determine the quantities consumed. The number of meals prepared during any day will depend on other labour demands on the time of the housewife, the amount of food available, the existence of other food sources (e.g. another kitchen in a polygamous household), the number and type of persons to be fed (remains of the previous night's supper may suffice for the children of the household but not for the household head) and perhaps the availability of fuel for cooking. After a hard day in the fields, the housewife may be too tired to prepare a family meal so she relies on food prepared in bulk which is consumed over a period of days. This is unhygienic and destroys precious vitamins. At such times of peak labour input when females as well as males are employed in the labour force, meals may be served too early or too late for non-work-force members. Young children may be in bed before the evening meal is prepared and if they remain in the village during the day may also go hungry at other times.

Methods of food allocation and meal sharing may have an even greater effect on food consumption levels than meal patterns. If the head of the family eats separately and is served first with the best food, other family members depend on what is left over. Food sharing may be more equal if the housewife serves individual members with what she considers to be their share but her rules for sharing may be based on custom rather than need. Common sense would suggest that available food is distributed to the workers rather than the non-work-force section but the village studies do not corroborate this. Anyway, even young children in poor families are employed and other unemployed but potential workers still need feeding in case they get jobs. Such effects probably vary with income levels, in that only the poorest families distribute food in relation to the earning potential of members. Options are removed when on-job feeding of agricultural labourers cuts out other family members from access to part of the income (i.e. the food) thus earned. It makes sense for the employer to pay his workers in 'calories', that is 'energy to do the job' but this could possibly result in the 'over-feeding' of adult males and more unequal distribution of food in already underfed families.

Eating from a common plate or self-service from a common pot benefits the fastest eaters and those of the family better co-ordinated to help themselves while the youngest child usually struggles to get his share (Food Science and Applied Nutrition Unit, 1968, p. 85). The presence of guests will divert even more food away from those members who do not partake in their entertaining especially if extra food is not prepared because it is unavailable or the guest was unexpected.

Dietary restrictions can exacerbate poor nutritional situations even if only spasmodically applied. Restrictions imposed upon an already sick and undernourished child can provoke a vicious cycle resulting in severe protein-calorie malnutrition. Other foods are tabooed because they are believed to affect behaviour patterns and others are forbidden for their supposed toxic effects. A diet rich in animal protein, for example, is believed in some Asian countries to make a mother's milk toxic to her breast-feeding infant but anyway, poor mothers often cannot afford such a diet. The direction of the effect of most food taboos can be evaluated but has not yet been quantified to the satisfaction of those alarmists among us who argue that malnutrition could be prevented if deleterious food taboos and habits were not practised.

The role of the housewife in the food distribution system is critical, the crucial elements being *decision making* and the *allocation of female time*. In subsistence villages where a year's supply of staples is often available only once-a-year, someone must decide how the food will be used over the whole year unless of course decisions are only made over a short period (Sharman, 1970). If some or all of the food is purchased, she must decide — if there is room for choice — how much of the total family income will be spent on food, and on what types of foods. Her decisions will affect the amount of food prepared for consumption in any one day, the number and timing of meals and sometimes how much each family member will consume. Amongst other things, she decides on the quantity of family food which the breadwinner will consume in the fields; the amounts the school-child will eat especially if he/she receives free school meals not available to other family members; the number of breast-feeds per day for the infant and the amount of money available for purchase of snacks by the pre-school child left on his own in the village while other family members are working.

Since the implications of these and other decision areas are serious for the nutritional status of family members, this is an obviously important area for new research. Another area is the *allocation* and *use* of female time, marginal differences in which may be partly responsible for intra- and inter-household variations in nutritional status. Female time and labour must be allocated between tasks as diverse as breast-feeding and weeding and the allocation of this time between all the different activities will affect both food availability, use of food and its distribution (Schofield, 1974b). Job allocation and labour utilisation vary between villages as cropping patterns, irrigation facilities, man—land ratios, etc. vary. We found that some jobs are performed by men and women together; others can be performed by either males or females but in general, there is for most jobs outside the domestic sphere, clear allocation by age and sex. Hipsley and Kirk (1965) found that in New Guinea, jobs were traditionally sex-linked. Male garden activities were found to include grass cutting, trenching and draining; planting; cultivating; harvesting and fencing, while women were mainly concerned with planting, harvesting and cultivation of specific crops. Unfortunately data on the different calorie costs of jobs are minimal and varied. Even so, female jobs such as weeding are often more time consuming and labour intensive than male jobs. Thus Haswell (1943) found that in a Gambian village, male farmers worked under 600 hours a year on crops and females under 1,110 hours.

Therefore, females also directly contribute to food availability in terms of their labour inputs in the agricultural sphere. However, their productivity will also vary with their food consumption: females whose calorie supply is insufficient to meet their energy demands will suffer the nutritional effects of an energy gap. The allocation of additional food to women involved in agricultural work will depend on whether males are simultaneously employed in heavy agricultural work, whether or not food is preferentially distributed to the work-force section of the population and whether it is distributed without sexual discrimination. Use of female time in energy demanding agricultural work without a corresponding increase in food supplies will affect female nutritional status. Those who will suffer most are the pregnant and lactating females who need more food to compensate for foetus growth and milk output but are not usually excluded from work in the fields. They and the foetus or young child will suffer in relation to the use of their time.

Type of use of female time directly affects female nutritional status (calories used in relation to those expended) and infant health. However, actual allocation of female time is another variable. Female labour time is allocated between agriculture and other activities such as food gathering, grain preparation, cooking, fuel and water collection; house-cleaning, etc. Chawdhuri found in a survey of 60 farm families that adult women spend more than half of their working hours on domestic chores in which 'preparation of meals, milling, fetching water and sweeping and washing dominate' while in the agricultural sector 'cattle and dairying take the lion's share of her energy' (1961, p. 648). However, the situation is not constant as seasonal agricultural demands such as harvesting, threshing, winnowing, weeding and planting and harvesting of sugar cane as well as gur making (Chawdhuri, 1961) will interrupt other activities. Women will have less time for the preparation of special infant foods and may have less energy to supervise family food distribution at meal times. Certain foods which have to be gathered, such as green leafy vegetables, may be omitted from the diet if the female is too busy with agricultural activities; quick, easy-to-prepare meals of nutritionally poorer staples such as cassava may be produced once a day or in bulk. In many areas where water carrying is traditionally a woman's job, females may have to spend up to four hours each day carrying home the family water supply from a distant well. If time is limited, the amount of water collected will be less and the frequency of bathing, laundering and floor washing, etc. will be reduced. Time constraints also inhibit house-cleaning, fuel collection (a water-boiling and cooking constraint) and child care which is especially important for the under-fives who have not built up resistance to many infections and are dependent on others for their food supply.

Aspects of child care, depending on age, include: all stages of feeding (breast feeding, supplementation, weaning and infant feeding); child hygiene which involves everything from washing to provision of clean clothes and toilet training; child supervision to prevent contact with sources of contamination (including other sick children); social training and education. Some have more important nutritional implications than others but they are all difficult to measure since assessment 'requires a value judgement which can only be made with an intimate knowledge of the mother—child relationship' (Desai, 1970, p. 141). Thus few surveys include such data. Huenemann (1954) in measuring the amount of time spent by each child with different child care agents in a Peruvian village was the exception. However, they did not assess the impact of child care on nutritional status.

Reallocation of responsibility for child care to siblings and other family members will depend on the type and size of family, work patterns, the time of year and the age of the child. For example, young breast-fed infants may either be taken to the fields or the mothers may return periodically to feed them. For older, weaned children, Antrobus (1971) found that those receiving day care from an adult were heavier and gained weight faster than those cared for mainly by a child. The siblings taking care of young dependants are sometimes not much older than the child and may also be participating in the work-force sector. Grandmothers generally perform child care functions better than siblings because they have had longer experience with young children and occupy a more stable economic position within the family.

Factors Affecting Seasonal Differences in Nutrition/Nutritional Status

Although factors affecting the year-round availability of food are numerous we have focused our attention on traditional subsistence villages dependent upon producing their own supplies of food and making these last throughout the year. Here small-holders, large-landowners, owners of small home-gardens and agricultural labourers (who are paid in produce as well as cash), all obtain some, most or all of their foods from subsistence production. We have ignored other food inputs into the village and the equalising effect of food storage facilities upon the year-round distribution of food. To some extent this has been forced upon us because most village nutrition studies do not include information on food storage and those that do, do not provide in-depth information. For example, they may describe the types of containers in which food is kept but give no data on how much is kept and for how long. General village studies provide better storage data (Coller, 1960).

However, we have already shown that seasonal differences in food consumption occur in villages and that these differences are more significant in mono-cropping, rain dependent villages with a uni-modal rainfall than continuous cropping villages with a bimodal distribution of rain. We have also cited individual examples to show how seasonal shortages are related to the socio-economic activities of the village.

Seasonal food shortages on their own are bad enough but what we have so far ignored are the other seasonality factors such as labour inputs and disease incidence which, when combined with seasonal food shortages, can really exacerbate the nutritional situation. The type, timing and intensity of village labour inputs determines the seasonal demand for energy and thus food. In subsistence villages subject to a well distributed rainfall, agricultural labour inputs are more likely to be evenly distributed throughout the year. Labour inputs will peak at different times of ploughing, planting, weeding and harvesting depending on type of crop and therefore types of related activities. These activities also have different calorie demands such that all labour peaks are not equally labour intensive and energy demanding. Thus the planting peak can be less labour intensive than the combined coincident activities of harvesting early food crops, sowing of late crops and weeding (Cleave, 1970) which all peak at the same time. Unfortunately, peak-season labour inputs often coincide with seasonal food shortages of the type described earlier. For example, Fox (1953) found that in Gambia, total energy expenditure exceeded food intake from June to October when agricultural activity was most intense and food inadequate. Collis found a similar situation in Nigeria and added that 'it is paradoxical that the people get more food at the time of year when they are less hard worked' (1962, p. 205).

The combined effect of heavy labour inputs and food shortages on nutritional status can lead to weight loss (as Bailey (1963) found in New Guinea), depletion of muscle tissue and impaired physical ability which can be worse for the more vulnerable sectors of the population. The body stores calories as body fat which accumulates in periods of food surplus, but post-harvest food surpluses do not always compensate for earlier food deficits as Gamble found in a Gambian village where 'an average of 60 per cent of calorie requirements is taken for six months of the year, February to July, and an average of 120 per cent of calorie requirements for only three months, mid-August to mid-November. Allowing an intermediate figure for the remaining four months, this would give an annual average of only 80 per cent of calorie requirements for adults' (Gamble, 1952, p. 18). Within villages, we cannot be sure which villagers are most affected by seasonal shortages in food. The small, subsistence farmer dependent on both family labour and his own farm-produced food is less likely to be able to afford to purchase extra food while large farmers can usually afford to import food staples but may not pay their agricultural labourers higher wages to compensate for higher food prices. This is because 'in developing economies wages often lag behind price rises and rural wages are notoriously slow in adjusting to rises in the cost of living. In periods when rural wages lag considerably behind price rises, agricultural labourers are bound to suffer, while landowners and entrepreneurs operate with an obvious advantage' (Epstein, 1975, p. 172). Similarly, we cannot be sure which persons in the family are most affected by seasonal shortages especially when females and young children are employed in the agricultural sector. The effect of food seasonalities and energy deficits (as labour inputs peak) on individuals will – to a certain extent – depend on the timing of male and female jobs and whether they are (a) employed at the same time and (b) simultaneously employed on tasks requiring a high energy output. Female labour use may be seasonal, as in a Gambian village where women worked almost exclusively on rice crops and men were occupied with groundnuts and millet (Haswell, 1943). Cleave (1970) argues that in Africa, 'at peak activity the men appear to work on crops no more than 30 hours a week, when planting and harvesting groundnuts. The urgency of harvesting swamp rice in January includes a 45-hour working week in the fields by the women. Apart from the differences in daily and total working hours it is noticeable that, within the limits of a nine-month agricultural season, the seasonal patterns of male and female work are completely different. In December and January when the women and working girls are most fully occupied, the men appear to have time on their hands. In September, the women spend three out of every four days clearing and planting the rice fields, but the men spend only seven days in the month in the field and under half of this time is spent helping with rice operations' (1970, p. 71).

However, the village studies do not tell us whether more food is given to all workers at times of peak labour demand. Are women fed when weeding and men when ploughing? In this case, common sense would suggest that available food is distributed to the workers such that the non-work-force section bears the brunt of seasonal variation in food supplies. If male and female seasonal labour inputs peak simultaneously, and males receive more than their fair share of food, male productivity levels will be maintained at the expense of female output. However, foregone production is not the only cost involved. Females have other tasks to perform which will get done in a haphazard fashion or not at all if other demands on their time and energy are high.

Seasonal food shortages, exacerbated by increasing seasonal requirements for food, can be worsened still further by the presence of infections and diseases. On their own, diseases can cause a deterioration in nutritional status (Scrimshaw, 1968) but if this is already impaired then effects could be far worse. Some of these diseases are also seasonally incident: diarrhoea occurs in all seasons, though it tends to peak when related to other infections (e.g. malaria and measles), and its lowest incidence is during the cold months. Pneumonia and bronchitis peak in cold weather; tuberculosis, measles, whooping cough and typhoid are more common in hot seasons and anaemia in the hot, wet seasons (Gordon, 1965).

However, the net effect of seasonal labour inputs, food shortages, the incidence of disease, food maldistribution and the possibility of extra consumption by adult males as their energy expenditure increases will have more detrimental effects on some individuals than others. Notably pregnant and lactating females whose condition does not entitle them to do less work. Indeed, pregnant women often work right up to the time of delivery. If maternal nutritional status is impaired by all these time and energy demands, so may the nutritional status of the baby. Here we shall consider both the indirect (via the mother) and direct effects of seasonality factors on the nutritional status of infants and children. Three groups of women are relevant: (a) pregnant women in the last trimester of pregnancy who give birth in the season of peak labour input or just after; (b) lactating females with infants aged from 0 to 6 months and (c) lactating females with infants over 6 months of age.

For group (a) mothers, a heavy energy expenditure when food is short could reduce the supply of food to the foetus and therefore affect the baby's birth weight depending on age and time of foetal weight gain. For example, in Nigeria, Morley (1968) found that the incidence of low-weight neonates is highest from January to June, after the January season of food scarcity and the beginning of the agricultural season in April; McGregor (1968) found the same phenomena in Gambia.

Infants of low birth weight are nutritionally more vulnerable to infections against which they have no active immunity and to nutritional deprivation from poor, inadequate or infrequent breast-feeding. The evidence suggests that babies with low birth weights are more likely to suffer continuous weight falterings. For example, Morley (1968) compared the weights and subsequent mortality of two groups of Nigerian infants (one with low and the other with high birth weights) and found that differences in birth weights between the two groups were related to their subsequent weight progress. Low birth weight babies are also likely to be less resistant to infections when passive immunity is lost at the age of 6 months. Evidence is, unfortunately, inconsistent. In the Gambia, McGregor (1968) found few, if any, definite associations between low birth weights and morbidity, and rate of weight gain could not be significantly correlated with morbidity. However, in the same country, Marsden (1965) found that weight faltering is associated with clinical illness. Although falterings are more common after 6 months, 15 of the 16 weight falterings from 0 to 6 months were caused by clinical illness. The relationship is reciprocal and cumulative since Morley (1968) argues that children underweight at 6–12 months are most likely to have suffered from measles or whooping cough in the first year.

For group (b) females, inadequate maternal diet accompanied by a heavy work load, may reduce milk output. Thomson (1967) substantiated this in a survey of a West African village where it was found that the pressures of farming and domestic work cause some women to cease lactating relatively early. These pressures may also affect the regularity of breast-feeding but this will depend on whether or not the child accompanies the mother to the fields or remains in the village. If left at home and in the absence of wet nurses, the child will not be breast-fed until the mother returns from work and will probably receive inadequate child care and feeding from employed nursemaids or siblings. On the other hand, if taken to the fields (e.g. rice swamps) with their mother, the infant may be more exposed to the seasonal incidence of infections than if they stay in the village since mosquito prevalence is higher in the rice swamps than the village.

In group (c), children are often breast-fed until 2 or more years of age. The quality and quantity of types of food supplementation are most important for this age group, but mothers with a heavy work-load will have less time to prepare and distribute food to the children. In total, infants, especially in the 0–24 month age group, are indirectly affected by the seasonality of female labour inputs through their effects on birth weights; the adequacy of breastfeeding/supplementary feeding and quality and quantity of child care; seasonal food shortages combined with the effects of intra-family maldistribution of foods (mainly in the 6 month plus age group); and the seasonal incidence of disease. The effects of these seasonal factors will vary with the age of the child and hence the birth season which determines the child's immediate (0–6 months) and future vulnerability to the effects of seasonality factors. In so far as passive immunity and breast-feeding protect infants from the seasonal effects of some diseases and food shortages at birth and for the first six months, the impact of seasonal factors will be greatest from 6 to 23 months. Birth season determines when passive immunity is lost so that children born six months before the season of peak disease incidence will be especially vulnerable to infection. Birth season will also affect weaning patterns (via the use of female time) and supplementation (in relation to seasonal food shortages).

We investigated the long-term effects of birth season in subsistence villages subject to the effects of one wet season and one dry season, each with two halves (e.g. first half of first dry season and second half of first dry season) and assume that female agricultural labour inputs peak in the wet season and are minimal in the dry season. Thus during the first two years of life, a child experiences the nutritional effects of four seasons (first dry season, first wet season, second dry season and second wet season), or eight half seasons. In tables 6.3 to 6.6, we investigate the long-term effects of births in different seasons: birth in the first half of the first dry season; birth in the second half of the first dry season; birth in the first half of the first wet season and birth in the second half of the first wet season. The long-term effects of birth season are measured by *birth-weight, breast-feeding, supplementary feeding, immunity and child care*. From our analysis of village study data we assume that:

1. birth-weight is 'good' in seasons of minimal female labour inputs,
2. breast-feeding is always 'limited' at periods of peak female labour input, and after 6 months of age when the amount of milk produced is insufficient to maintain adequate growth without proper supplementation,

Table 6.3: Effects of Seasonality of Birth on the Nutritional Status of Pre-School Children. Birth in the First Half of the First Dry Season

	First Dry Season (D)		First Wet Season (W)		Second Dry Season (2D)		Second Wet Season (2W)	
	First Half of First Dry Season D_1	Second Half of First Dry Season D_2	First Half of First Wet Season W_1	Second Half of First Wet Season W_2	First Half of Second Dry Season $2D_1$	Second Half of Second Dry Season $2D_2$	First Half of Second Wet Season $2W_1$	Second Half of Second Wet Season $2W_2$
Age of child	0–3m.	4–6m.	7–9m.	10–12m.	13–15m.	16–18m.	19–21m.	22–24m.
Birth weight	Good	–	–	–	–	–	–	–
Breast-feeding	Unlimited	Unlimited	Limited	Limited	Limited	Limited	Limited	Limited
Supplementary feeding	–	–	Limited	Limited	Unlimited	Unlimited	Limited	Limited
Type of immunity	Passive	Passive	No immunity to wet season diseases	No immunity to wet season diseases	No immunity to dry season diseases	No immunity to dry season diseases	Active	Active
Child care	Good	Good	Limited	Limited	Good	Good	Limited	Limited

Table 6.4. Birth in the Second Half of the First Dry Season

	First Dry Season (D)		First Wet Season (W)		Second Dry Season (2D)		Second Wet Season (2W)		Third Dry Season (3D)
	D_1	D_2	W_1	W_2	$2D_1$	$2D_2$	$2W_1$	$2W_2$	$3D_1$
Age of child	—	0–3m.	4–6m.	7–9m.	10–12m.	13–15m.	16–18m.	19–21m.	22–24m.
Birth weight	—	Good	—	—	—	—	—	—	—
Breast-feeding	—	Unlimited	Limited	Limited	Limited	Limited	Limited	Limited	Limited
Supplementary feeding	—	—	—	Limited	Unlimited	Unlimited	Limited	Limited	Unlimited
Type of immunity	—	Passive	Passive	No immunity to wet season diseases	No immunity to dry season diseases	No immunity to dry season diseases	Active	Active	Active
Child care	—	Good	Limited	Limited	Good	Good	Limited	Limited	Good

Table 6.5: Birth in the First Half of the First Wet Season

	First Wet Season (W)		First Dry Season (D)		Second Wet Season (2W)		Second Dry Season (2D)	
	W_1	W_2	D_1	D_2	$2W_1$	$2W_2$	$2D_1$	$2D_2$
Age of child	0–3m.	4–6m.	7–9m.	10–12m.	13–15m.	16–18m.	19–21m.	22–24m.
Birth weight	Low	–	–	–	–	–	–	–
Breast feeding	Limited	Limited	Limited	Limited	Limited	Limited	Limited	Limited
Supplementary feeding	–	–	Unlimited	Unlimited	Limited	Limited	Unlimited	Unlimited
Type of immunity	Passive	Passive	No immu- to dry season diseases	No immu- to dry season diseases	No immu- to wet season diseases	No immu- to wet season diseases	Active	Active
Child care	Limited	Limited	Good	Good	Limited	Limited	Good	Good

Table 6.6: Birth in the Second Half of the First Wet Season

	First Wet Season (W)		First Dry Season (D)		Second Wet Season (2W)		Second Dry Season (2D)		Third Wet Season (3W)
	W_1	W_2	D_1	D_2	$2W_1$	$2W_2$	$2D_1$	$2D_2$	$3W_1$
Age of child	–	0–3m.	4–6m.	7–9m.	10–12m.	13–15m.	16–18m.	19–21m.	22–24m.
Birth weight	–	Low	–	–	–	–	–	–	–
Breast-feeding	–	Limited	Unlimited	Limited	Limited	Limited	Limited	Limited	Limited
Supplementary feeding	–	–	–	Unlimited	Limited	Limited	Unlimited	Unlimited	Limited
Type of immunity	–	Passive	Passive	No immunity to dry season diseases	No immunity to wet season diseases	No immunity to wet season diseases	Active	Active	Active
Child care	–	Limited	Good	Good	Limited	Limited	Good	Good	Limited

3. supplementary feeding is 'limited' in the season of food shortages and peak family labour inputs,
4. immunity is 'passive' for a period of 6 months after birth, while immunity is 'active' only after exposure to infection, say 12–18 months after birth, and
5. child care other than feeding (e.g. general supervision, bathing, etc.) is 'limited' when agricultural labour inputs are high.

Table 6.7 summarises the effects of all those factors on the vulnerability of children from birth to 24 months of age. However, without giving each birth season a numerical weighting, which at best would be somewhat arbitrary, we cannot reliably conclude that in this hypothetical situation there is a 'best' season for births. Children born in any season will, at some stage in the first two years of life, be vulnerable to the effects of seasonality factors. Children born in the first half of the first dry season will be very vulnerable at 7–12 months of age; those born in the second half of the first dry season will be relatively vulnerable at 7–18 months of age; those born in the first half of the first wet season will be vulnerable at birth and from 16 to 18 months of age while those born in the second half of the first wet season will be vulnerable at 24 months of age.

Table 6.7: Vulnerability of Different Age Groups Dependent on Birth Season

Age	Most Vulnerable to the Effects of Seasonal Factors		Least Vulnerable to the Effects of Seasonal Factors	
	Birth season			
Birth	W_1	W_2	D_2	D_1
7–12m.	D_1	D_2	W_2	W_1
16–18m.	W_1	D_2	D_1	W_2
24m.	W_2 D_1	—	—	D_2 W_1

The implications of this analysis will ultimately depend on the age at which vulnerability to seasonal factors is most crucial. If vulnerability is most critical at birth, then children born in the first half of the first dry season are best off; if vulnerability is more critical at 7–12 months of age when passive immunity is lost and breast-feeding becomes inadequate, then children born in the first half of the first wet season will be least vulnerable here; at 16–18 months of age, children born in the second half of the first wet season will be best off and at 24 months of age, children born either in the second half of the first dry season or the first half of the first wet season will be least vulnerable.

To minimise the effects of seasonality, nutrition intervention should also be seasonal and targeted at the age groups of children who are most vulnerable. Demographic studies showing the seasons at which births peak could help. For example, Gamble (1952) shows that in the Gambia Protectorate, births peak in August and September whereas in a three year demographic study in Bangladesh, Chowdhury and others (1970) found October—December birth peaks which coincide with peak labour inputs and food shortages.

Conclusions

Village data, limited though they are, provide evidence of intra-village differences in food and nutrient intake levels especially between occupational and income groups. These suggest that households at different income levels may require separate and different nutrition intervention programmes. The studies also point to the need for identifying simple socio-economic indicators which can be used by clinic or other staff for detecting families at social risk of malnutrition.

Problems of food supply within the village are just one aspect of the problem of undernutrition. Within the family, other factors affect the quality and quantity of foods consumed by individuals and cause intra-household differences in nutritional status. We are concerned with the pattern of food/nutrient distribution between parents, notably adult males, and children. The village data indicate that sex selective child feeding and the distribution of food between family workers are essential research areas. If total food is insufficient, emphasis on better family distribution, to respect the requirements of all rather than a few family members, is a must for nutrition education schemes unless there is a definite rationale for providing working male adults with more of the family food. When diversion of food from the male to other family members leads to reduced productivity, the costs of supplementary feeding may be inescapable. At best, food could be redistributed to meet the additional seasonal work demands of all sectors of the population.

Use and allocation of female time is another area for research. Provision of food supplements should be considered within the time constraints of the poorer village mother. Has she time to prepare the supplementary food, and is she available to collect it at the hour, day and season of distribution? Lack of labour time or of cash may be equally important in preventing adoption of such health practices as boiling water. New projects like home gardens, which further constrain female time, will be less effective than other inputs such as provision of water carrying trolleys which attempt to alleviate time constraints.

The effects of seasonal factors must also be taken into consideration when planning programmes since they have policy implications both for timing and type of improvement or prevention programme. In villages with a single rainy season, provision of adequate storage facilities may do more for nutrition than food supplementation from external sources. Supplementation programmes should be seasonal, operating at times of peak labour input. Special programmes for vulnerable groups, including pregnant or lactating women, will also benefit unborn infants and breast-fed children. Mothers, given adequate supplementary feeding, should be advised to breast-feed as long as possible, partly in the hope of delaying conception and creating longer birth intervals, but mainly to compensate food shortages. Night-feeding of infants, especially where work demands prevent regular daily breast-feeding, and prevention of weaning in the hot season when supplementary foods deteriorate quickly, should also be encouraged. Peak disease incidence in any season should direct the timing of immunisation and other preventive schemes along with the timing of curative programmes. Timing of prevention schemes should of course also be determined by the age of the child. Family planning services could include advice on the timing of conception to minimise the risk of birth in disadvantageous seasons. If birth peaks are clear-cut, other nutrition and health education programmes should be initiated before birth peaks to educate women on the hygiene of child-birth, methods of supplementation, etc. This will be successful only if birth peaks do not coincide with peak labour inputs when women may have no time to participate in nutrition programmes. There is conflict here in that mothers have time for programmes in the dry season but their infants need the protection these programmes could provide during the wet season. This conflict may be resolved by the provision of seasonal day care or pre-school centres. Scarce staff resources may be best utilised for seasonal, perhaps mobile centres in the rainy season and for education programmes in the dry season as in Taiwan, where in addition to the permanent rural day care centres, seasonal day care nurseries were provided for children whose mothers work in the rice fields (UNICEF, 1967).

7 IMPLEMENTATION OF NUTRITION PROGRAMMES AT THE MICRO LEVEL

So far we have shown how micro-level studies aid identification and classification of nutrition problems so that planners can (a) evaluate the types of programmes that would most benefit any local community, (b) assess the felt village 'needs', (c) time programme implementation to fit in with village work patterns, and (d) evaluate the probable effectiveness of development programmes before introduction. Village studies can also help us to understand why development programmes are rejected or accepted at the micro level by isolating all the factors which are either (a) prohibitive or (b) conducive to successful programme implementation. They also illuminate how programmes could be better organised to fit in more successfully with the village way of life.

Choice of Relevant Programmes and Village Needs

Efforts to reach villages with improvement programmes are often part of a national blanket programme which ignores individual village needs. Thus regional latrine programmes are implemented in villages with an inadequate water supply and village soakage pits unsuccessfully introduced to villages whose soil was unsuitable for that type of construction. Such programmes need to be modified (Learmonth, 1962) to suit village needs and conditions and this is where we hope the classificatory approach to village problems could be usefully employed. We feel that other VSP advice is relevant here for although some villages may need specific programmes, the projected response to new innovations may influence the way they are implemented or may determine whether or not they are worthwhile implementing in relation to accrued benefits. For instance, certain communities may respond better to community rather than individually oriented programmes; to innovations particularly in agriculture which do not require a lot of risk taking; to programmes with quick and visible effects such as DDT spraying to eradicate mosquitoes, or to projects which provide villages with a clear-cut idea of the types of benefits they are likely to receive compared with programmes that do not. For example, programmes aimed at increasing agricultural output have clearer benefits than village welfare projects whose aims are less visible. In Uttar Pradesh it was found that although the public health and sanitation programmes 'touched a very considerable proportion of village people ... they were not pushed forward with the urgency and

112

enthusiasm that were shown in the agricultural extension programme' (Dube, 1958, p. 70).

Our second piece of advice is that in order to avoid detracting efforts from the most essential elements of a programme, the objectives should be limited and clearly defined. In one Indian village (Dube, 1955), the auxiliary projects (a clinic, social nights, chicken coop and pig breeding programmes) only served to confuse public understanding of the specific goal of the programme which was to establish a school feeding programme. We also believe that planners and administrators should always consult those government agents best acquainted with the villages to which resources will be allocated. Assessment of the innovations most essential for improving the quality of village life (electricity for one village, irrigation for another and wells for a third) must be based on the 'felt village needs'. These should be familiar to the village worker but would take any other person unfamiliar with the village some time to perceive. Any programme which contradicts these needs is in danger of jeopardy. For example, Fraser (1968, p. 395) describes how a village level worker was unsuccessful in disseminating nutritional information and knowledge about safe water supplies because the villagers were only interested in programmes bringing medical care into the village.

Lastly, it is essential to study the timing of programmes which should fit in with the sometimes inflexible demands of the village work calendar. For example, Khare (1964) describes how, in India, DDT spraying was successful because it was completed in the slack agricultural season. Similarly, one of the reasons for the success of the Indian Barpali vegetable growing programme (Fraser, 1968) was the fact that these activities were initiated in the two slack periods (1) between the initial planting and harvesting of rice, and (2) in the post-harvest period. Choice of timing is not always so clear-cut: Fraser states that in India it is easier to install latrines in the dry season because cave-ins are less likely but unfortunately 'this season presents fewest problems which might be eased by the use of latrines' (1963, p. 87). It is better — in terms of getting people to accept these innovations — to install them in the rainy season because people are reluctant to visit distant and muddy fields when conditions are generally uncomfortable. However, education programmes will probably have more impact if introduced during the slack dry season while other programmes such as seasonally operating day care centres could be introduced during the wet season to alleviate the effects of seasonal factors at times of peak female agricultural labour inputs. Preventive immunisation schemes should be timed well before the season of peak disease incidence and curative programmes (e.g. the distribution of iron tablets) should also be timed for periods of peak need (maximum anaemia incidence).

Village Variables Prohibitive to Development Programmes

All societies are based on an integrated system of relationships and institutions which are structured and meaningful to the members of the society. Any new innovation will impinge on this highly ordered system by adding to it or replacing old elements. In the former case the better it is adapted to the existing system, the fewer the number of conflicts. Sometimes conflict is inevitable; but outsiders seeking to replace old elements (e.g. village money-lenders) will need to ask if such elements fulfilled a real need, and if so, fulfil it also in the new relationships. Only through micro-level studies can we isolate those factors that are likely to be prohibitive or conducive to programme implementation. Here we will discuss social, political and economic factors and cultural systems as they effect the implementation of nutrition intervention programmes and other related programmes with an indirect effect on nutritional levels.

Social, Political and Economic Factors

It is generally believed that villagers are co-operative and work together for community ends. But traditionally villagers co-operate by accepting and maintaining reciprocal obligations rather than working together for community goals: Thus programmes based on communal activity are implemented under a misconception: to introduce community orchards and co-operative tractor ownership where farms are traditionally owned by close groups of kin and there is no communal action at the village level is a waste of time.

This was recognised by Lewis (1955) who saw that the one mistake in the introduction of a medical clinic to a Mexican village was its organisation on a co-operative basis, because a long standing co-operative tradition was lacking. The implications for communally operated nutrition programmes within similar types of village are the same. Communal village gardens to provide vegetables and other supplementary foods for the village may be equally doomed to failure.

Outsiders, such as extension agents, come into the village and ask for or expect the co-operation of the villagers in order to instigate development projects. This behaviour may again be foreign to villages since leaders within the village obtain a following, and therefore co-operation, not by virtue of their status but by fulfilling obligations (F. G. Bailey, 1969). Behaviour outside village norms will either be humorous to the villagers or cause them to worry and will certainly constrain the acceptance of nutrition programmes based on village co-operation. Extension agents, village level workers, or any other outsider entering a village 'must recognise the implications of the fact that they are not entering a power vacuum' (Lewis, 1955, p. 431) but impinging upon a complex network of relationships. New institutions may be rejected because they upset the balance of power within a village and because those involved want to maintain the existing system of relationships. Lewis (1955) shows how the leading medical prac- titioner in a Mexican village saw the medical co-operative as a power threat because no group could claim credit for its introduction and it served as a reminder of how little the officials did for the village.

The people, institutions and structures that make and implement decisions on behalf of the community such as the co-operative societies, schools, and above all, the village council or panchayat should not be alienated by programmes or their administrators. For example, Oberg and Rios (1955) describe the organisation and implementation of agricultural, health and educational services directed at the small Brazilian village of Chonin de Cina. A community council was formed which was intended by the programme planners as a device for involving the community. However, the committee chairman chosen for the council was a member of the party which was out of power in the district and this alienated the local group in office from the project. Khare (1964) describes how in an Indian village the vaccinator was attacked, not because the villagers distrusted the injections and rejected the programme but because he had quarrelled with a village leader.

Formalised structures may not be the only power base in traditional villages; other informal but authoritative structures exist and function successfully because they operate through moral sanctions. Efforts to provide a pre-paid medical service in Barpali Thana (Fraser, 1968) failed because they were directed through the gram panchayats (the regional governing councils), which were not really functioning as part of the social structure and did not reflect the real patterns of power, authority and leadership. Faction leaders are especially important and project organisers must acquaint themselves with the membership of village factions and identify and contact their leaders. Factions are primarily kinship units rather than political groupings but their presence can be both prohibitive and conducive to development work. They have important social, economic and ceremonial functions and also act as cohesive units in opposition to other castes when the opportunity arises as at court litigations and elections. Factions will deter programme implementation if acceptance of a development goal by one faction automatically leads to its rejection by the opposing faction (e.g. the acceptance of latrines). The opposition between factions can also provide an excuse for failure to implement programmes as each faction accuses the other for failing to reach the desired goals concerning the improvement of village conditions.

Self-interested groups such as castes, a feature peculiar to Indian society, can affect the success of development programmes. Membership is by birth and confers a ritual status on a rigid hierarchical system. Castes are endogamous and have exclusive commensal relations with and specific duties to others. Members of the same caste often live in the same quarter of the village, specialise in one occupation, eat the same foods, and avoid certain types of contact such as eating with or drinking from the same source as members of other castes.

The effect of caste divisions on the acceptance of development programmes is not clear-cut but will depend on the type of programme. The idea of ritual pollution between castes by eating, socialising and physical contact is especially important for nutritional and sanitation programmes. Thus Moffatt (1974) found that locating the Balwady infant feeding programme in the Harijan colony, traditionally located on the outskirts of the village, prohibited participation by Caste Hindus. The optimum location was found to be half-way between the village and the colony. He also found that a Harijan Balasevika is acceptable but a Harijan Ayya is not and the food will not be received by the upper castes if cooked in the colony. Similarly, Dube (1958) describes how the presence of female Untouchables in the education classes resulted in a boycott by the upper caste women: this has obvious implications for nutrition education.

One aspect of Sanskritisation is that the lower castes try to emulate the upper castes by obtaining ritually purer jobs. However, this factor of job status can be detrimental for development efforts as Fraser (1968) shows in a description of an attempt to improve nutritional standards through the introduction of better quality poultry. The poultry scheme was rejected by the lower castes because they did not want to increase their involvement in an occupation held to be ritually inferior, as this might reduce their possibility of upward mobility. Those who did adopt poultry raising were found to be members of the upper caste who looked upon it as a business instead of an occupation.

Other socio-economic divisions within the village are primarily based on the ownership or non-ownership of the means of production which is land in rural areas. These inequalities in the distribution of wealth and power have obvious repercussions for the distribution of the effects of development programmes. Those who 'have nothing to begin with, nothing which can be improved, no means of getting an economic start' (Mandelbaum, 1955, p. 18) have nothing to lose with improvement programmes. Similarly, they often have nothing to gain as many programmes (e.g. irrigation and mechanisation schemes, the introduction of new seeds) function primarily to improve agricultural productivity which benefits the farmers and landowners but is of no immediate benefit to the agricultural labourers. With nothing to gain, they will hardly be willing to co-operate in order to increase the advantages which the farmers already enjoy. Similarly, general programmes in the field of sanitation and public health often have less relevance to the lives of the poorer sections of the community who are pre-occupied with achieving subsistence. With the mobilisation of Shramdan (free) labour for village co-operative work the upper castes assume a managerial role while the lower castes are left to do all the work. Traditional work patterns are once more reinforced and the labourers receive no payment and simultaneously have to forfeit the income they could be earning elsewhere.

There are two problems here. First, an approach which ignores differences in socio-economic position, motivations and attitudes and which insists on dealing with the village as a unit for all development programmes, may well lead to a solidifying of economic and political positions within the caste hierarchy (Mencher, 1970, p. 216). Second, if we attempt to compensate for these differences by selective pro- grammes, structural divisions may be strengthened even further by virtue of opposition from the non-recipients. Either we (a) choose only those programmes that will benefit the entire population rather than small segments or we (b) make special efforts to ensure that the benefits of programmes are equally distributed among all the classes of a community or (c) select separate and different innovations and programmes for each group depending on their need or (d) attempt some combination of these. For example, (a) clinical facilities are demanded by rich and poor alike and provision of these will obviously receive wider village support than programmes benefiting only a select minority of the villagers. However, (b) we may still need special education programmes to ensure that poor backward families utilise the new medical facilities. An alternative may be to make these facilities available but to (c) introduce supplementary programmes for the special needs of the Harijan community who are usually worse off than the remainder of the population. Unfortunately, selective caste programmes may be viewed with suspicion by other castes and may further strengthen existing divisions within the village.

Another lesson to be learnt here is that village extension workers should not identify themselves with any particular group in the village. If they identify with the minority group, the majority of villagers may become somewhat indifferent or even hostile to them and the activities they advocate. Dube (1958) found this in India and Adams (1935) found that in a Guatemalan nutrition project, the social worker had become closely associated with one Barrio. As she made friends there, she became simultaneously less acceptable to the other.

The behaviour of the extension agent, village level worker, government official or project team and their relationships with the villagers is not received at its face value for two reasons. Firstly, people coming from outside the village usually have no ties of kinship or caste and therefore no structural means of being incorporated into the social order and secondly, outsiders are beyond the moral community of the village and are 'dangerous and sinful' (F. G. Bailey, 1969, p. 3). Villagers often expect that contracts made by outsiders will not be fulfilled and to ensure against this, villagers may practise 'anticipatory cheating'. Because extension agents are outside the moral community they are not expected to conform to village values and are often accused of being self-motivated, of running programmes mainly for the benefit of the organising agent and are accused of utilising projects, funds, medicines, etc. for their own ends. In some cases (Oberg and Rios, 1955, p. 367) extension agents manipulate the different political factions and play them off one against the other in order to achieve a powerful position. Behaviour of innovators is often colonial and patronising since they believe that other cultural groups are backward. superstitious and ignorant. Such attitudes are hardly conducive to co-operation.

In small-scale, face-to-face societies, relationships are multiplex with individuals assuming many roles. If new roles are introduced by extension agents, these must adapt to the inherent role system. Failure to do so will result in confusion and possible rejection. Thus when Dube was examining the impact of the Community Development programme in two villages of the Western Uttar Pradesh Community Project Block, he found that the villagers could not understand the role of the new midwife. 'Traditionally they could distinguish between the role of a trained doctor, and of an untrained village dai who assisted at childbirths. The role of the midwife, who was something between the two, was new to the village people. Because of her official position, clean clothes, and sophisticated language, village women at first regarded the midwife as a qualified doctor, and expected modern medical treatment and injections from her. Many of them were disillusioned when they discovered that she was neither trained nor officially permitted to do this. They hesitated in calling her to assist at childbirths, because, unlike the village dais, she refused to do any cleaning, and would not massage the mother and the baby in the weeks following the birth. For this they had to hire an untrained village dai' (1958, p. 75). Similarly, Western or Western trained doctors do not behave in the same way as local practitioners who are expected to have 'superior knowledge' of the body; they do not arrive at a diagnosis by asking questions about symptoms and they practise medicine for the sake of enhancing their own religious merit. In comparison, the Western doctor is an outsider who treats patients with an egalitarian attitude, sees the patient alone in a private interview without his family to support him and asks questions about the illness in order to arrive at a diagnosis. Rather than provide medicine direct, they give prescriptions which indicates to the villager that he is not skilled in their preparation and he usually requires payment for the treatment before its success has been proven.

People who are not respected by the villagers, e.g. unmarried women and widows without children, make unsuccessful agents. Respect and position are a help as Moffat found in comparing the running of a school lunch programme by the headmaster with the administration of the Balwady by the Balasevika. The headmaster manages the school lunch more efficiently because he can choose participants on a poverty basis; he knows the economic levels of the villagers and has enough prestige and standing not to succumb to local pressure for accepting better-off children. In comparison, the Balasevika and the Ayya had less success because they lacked prestige and were less immune to local pressure to accept children who were not eligible.

Programmes that interfere with traditional systems and try to change them are also likely to fail. Thus we can persuade Indian villagers to dig compost pits outside the village but purdah and other restrictions will prevent the women (traditional removers of garbage and cow-dung) from taking it outside the village. Labour intensive programmes or those requiring additional effort from overworked villagers will also be unpopular and this is the main reason for the failure of the latrine programme in Barpali village (Fraser, 1968). Every time the toilet was used it needed to be flushed with about a quart of water representing a daily additional water requirement of several gallons. Water carrying was a female occupation and they strongly resisted the idea of having to fetch and carry several more gallons of water per day. Similarly, women resist water boiling innovations because they simply have not got the time to do it (Wellin, 1955). Alternatively, they may make the time for new innovations by abandoning breast-feeding or adopting other innovations (polished rice) which may have even worse effects on health than drinking unboiled water.

Cultural System

One of the communal aspects of a village is the existence of a common set of standards, beliefs, values and norms of behaviour which are referred to by individuals deciding whether or not to innovate. Because people need support for their actions they will tend to behave like other community members within their own cultural structure. If they do not, it threatens the stability of social relationships, and the validity of communal values. These are often ignored by outsiders coming into the village who egoistically assume that their aims and means are convergent with those of the society they are attempting to improve and fail to understand the cultural system on which they are imposing. Local belief systems in particular are often dismissed as irrational superstitions. In reality however, beliefs form a coherent system which provides explanations for events otherwise beyond the scientific comprehension of many societies. Sometimes the rationale behind certain beliefs is apparent: for example, diets of pregnant women are restricted because people believe that this will ensure a small baby and easy delivery. Other beliefs such as ritual pollution of upper castes by lower caste members are less easy to comprehend. What is fundamental, however, is that beliefs in the separate spheres of religion, health, food, etc. are all interrelated to form a closed system within which failures can be explained. Thus, the failure of folk medicine is accepted because the patient was beyond help whereas the failure of a doctor to treat and cure a symptom cannot be accepted and the villagers will lose faith in him.

Since food and especially the struggle to provide enough food is an issue central to many cultures, especially to subsistence economies, all cultures have built up a series of traditional beliefs and attitudes towards food which are usually well entrenched. Restrictions on the use of food are common and relate to their use at certain times of the year (e.g. some foods are especially reserved for consumption at festivals) and by certain people: menstruating, pregnant and lactating women are a common focus of dietary restrictions, as are children. Many of these prohibitions relate to beliefs about the inherent nature of foods such as its 'hotness' or 'coldness' which is unrelated to its physical temperature. Foods may also be 'light' or 'heavy' or produce physical symptoms such as diarrhoea, constipation or worms. Some foods are believed to affect behaviour (eggs cause children to steal) while some physical illnesses are attributed to eating the wrong types of food. Some food practices are deleterious to health as when the withdrawal of milk and solid foods from the diet of a child suffering from diarrhoea precipitates severe protein-calorie deficiency. However, not all food beliefs are bad for the health and we must recognise differences between stated beliefs and practices. We must also distinguish between traditions and beliefs. Even though villagers do not believe that vegetables are bad for health they may not traditionally form part of the diet and therefore vegetable cultivation will be difficult to introduce. Similarly if peas are traditionally eaten by animals it may be difficult to try introducing improved types of peas. If such traditions are so hard to change then belief systems may be even more impervious.

By studying food habits, nutritionists or social scientists can evaluate the impact of current practices on nutritional status and determine points of intervention. Innovations which require beliefs to change will be less readily accepted than 'neutral', non-interfering programmes or ones that uphold traditional belief systems. Examples not directly involving nutrition include programmes interfering with traditional beliefs about ritual pollution: schemes to clean-up villages are abandoned by upper castes who fear pollution from contact with the polluting excreta of lower castes; drainage schemes can be ruled out if members of ritually polluting castes live near each other, while adoption of latrines is prohibited by the fact that latrines have to be located in or near the house where food is prepared.

Thus the success of any programme may depend on how radical or reformist the programme is. But in general, 'there is no propaganda agent so effective as a demonstrable cure' (Carstairs, 1955, p. 118). Villagers can accept successful cures which they cannot understand so long as they do not interfere with the belief system. For example, Dube found that the significance of malaria control 'was not understood by most of the people' (1958, p. 74) but because it was novel and they thought it 'improved the air' the practice was accepted. But if we cannot persuade the villager about the proper cause of the cure he may attribute it to a supernatural agent rather than the drug or injection. This partial adoption of new ideas may ensure incorporation of the new programme but can be dangerous if villagers for example believe that vaccinations need only be given once in a lifetime and that too at an early age so that secondary vaccinations are not easily accepted. Thus programmes should be carefully analysed to determine what part they would play in established systems. Perhaps after all, as Mead (1962) suggests, we should measure how food habits change before we can attempt to change them.

Village Variables Conducive to the Successful Implementation of Development Programmes

Although villages are often tied to tradition 'one must be constantly on one's guard against any naive assumption that whatever is traditional is *ipso facto* hostile to change' (Ishwaran, 1970b, p. 7). Village societies are never static entities and their potential for change could be utilised as a positive force. Groups within the village may have different attitudes towards programme proposals and if approached in the right way, Government officials may be able to get the support of at least one group. In India, the highly structured organisation of caste hierarchies can be made use of in programme implementation. The different foci of caste groups (some are more concerned with agriculture, education or goals outside the village), could provide useful starting points for development programmes while their inter-village organisation provides an ideal basis for the diffusion of innovations. Similarly, factions provide ready made groups and communication channels (Lewis, 1954, p. 36) for co-operative ventures, and, at the risk of sounding colonial, hostility between factions can be exploited in order to achieve development goals for their own good. Fraser (1968) describes a village in which there were two factions of nearly equal strength but whose leaders could not agree on the site for a new well. They finally decided to dig two wells at opposite ends of the village and there was serious competition to see which faction would finish first. Without this competition, the village would probably not have got the new well. Similarly, support of two different medical schemes (Barpali village services scheme and the government medical scheme) by two opposing factions ensured widespread village support for the introduction of improvements.

Within the village, authoritative and charismatic personalities should always be approached since programme successes often result from the efforts of local leaders whose personalities and abilities overcome cleavages within the village and outweigh frictions of caste, class, faction or religion. They may be able to persuade people to adopt innovations, such as latrines but unless they themselves are known to use the innovations (e.g. the new seeds), they may not be able to convince others.

Programmes may be accepted for reasons uncomplementary to the primary aims of the programme: prestigious items will be more quickly adopted than less prestigious ones (e.g. latrines or hand pumps). Fraser found that it was impossible to explain the scientific advantages of a protected water supply and that one Indian village accepted the intro- duction of wells not as a source of protected water but as an adequate supply of water. The village women had to walk more than half a mile to the village tank and even further to the river-bed if the tank was dry (Fraser, 1963). Thus a well in the middle of the village was not only convenient but ensured a continuous supply of water. 'Had the existing water resources of the area been sufficient for convenient use by every- one, a protected supply of water would not have made any progress at all' (1968, p. 227—8). Similarly, the vegetable programme was accepted as an alternative income source rather than as a new food source for improving nutritional levels. Traditionally, vegetables hardly had any place in the diet of Barpali villagers and efforts over two years to increase the quality and quantity of vegetables grown were not successful until a drought threatened to destroy the rice crop. As they became more important as a cash crop, increasing quantities were grown.

Thus the gloomy picture we presented earlier about the difficulties in programme implementation is not always accurate since programmes are accepted by villagers for a variety of reasons. But what we need to get is an overall picture of why they are accepted so that future pro- gramme implementation can become a science instead of an haphazard process.

Conclusions

Improvement programmes should be implemented in relation to specific needs. Even so, their success or failure may depend on village variables which we have discussed in this chapter. Unfortunately the success of nutrition programmes is rarely evaluated in terms of socio-economic factors and therefore we had to use evidence from studies of agricultural extension programmes, welfare projects and health programmes to illuminate the problems involved. Since (a) many development programmes have an impact in the nutritional sector; (b) nutritional and other programmes (e.g. health) have certain organisational and administrative features in common and (c) programmes and extension workers are often multi-purpose, we feel justified in quoting from these other case studies, and hope we have illuminated some of the problems involved.

Many programmes fail through inefficient project administration (Oberg and Rios, 1955), the organisational form of the project (Paul, 1955), the methods of policy making and the lack of organisational goals. These problems have not been discussed here as they are not specific to village studies. Instead we have discussed factors in the social, cultural, economic and political structure of the village that are prohibitive to development programmes. We have attempted to show some of the mistakes to be avoided and to indicate the types of sociological and anthropological information needed by village nutrition workers. Problems inherent in social relationships should be addressed cautiously and with conscious awareness of different cultural response patterns. Agents should approach groups whose solidarity will enable members to co-operate in new innovations and campaigns need to enlist the support of influential persons who must be identified with care in villages with a weak leadership and numerous factional groups.

8 CONCLUSIONS

No one today doubts that malnutrition exists. Even the 'man in the street' is aware of famines in Ethiopia, Bangladesh or any other less-developed country suddenly hit by floods, crop failure, drought or other extreme conditions conducive to famine. What both he and the experts are less aware of is the extent of the mild and moderate forms of malnutrition. Throughout the world, there is a general lack of data on the incidence of deficiency diseases because true random samples of populations are rarely surveyed and under-recording of the marginal cases of malnutrition is a severe problem. However, available literature indicates that protein calorie malnutrition is widespread, the incidence of anaemia is high and Vitamin A deficiencies severe. These occur throughout the world while other deficiencies are specific to particular areas. Mortality statistics, especially infant death rates, are particularly disturbing and indicative not only of nutritional deficiencies but of a high disease incidence as well.

Without an adequate diet, the quality of life is immediately and sometimes permanently impaired; people cannot earn a living, are mentally and physically impeded and are more susceptible to illness. One solution to the problem — rather negative because it involves no immediate action — is to let economic growth take care of all nutritional problems. Admittedly poverty is the prime cause of most malnutrition, but there are still several reasons for more immediate action. First, malnutrition impedes economic growth. Second, even in countries whose national incomes have risen, economic growth is rarely immediately reflected in income increments for the poor who are both economically and nutritionally worst off. Third, economic development policies which should eventually improve nutrition often in fact have the unintended side effect of causing malnutrition in some sectors of the population. Fourth, all human suffering must be alleviated as soon as possible by short-term measures.

Planners have to choose between non-nutrition oriented programmes such as income redistribution schemes and measures to improve employment and rural productivity and programmes which have a direct effect on nutrition such as diet supplementation. The former however require a massive policy reformulation and have more political implications than direct action. Therefore the real choice is between blanket and specific action programmes. Blanket programmes achieve maximum coverage but these are sometimes wasteful, since in order to solve the nutrition problems of those in need they also cover large numbers of people not in need of the extra nutrients, food or help. What is needed are more programmes to meet specific nutritional needs. However, we cannot systematically plan to achieve this until we can successfully identify nutritional problems.

Nutritional deficiencies are usually identified by type (PCM or Vitamin A deficiency), size (percentage of the population affected) and location. Nutritionally at risk areas in types of ecological zone or typically vulnerable groups have been selected but not by any systematic classificatory system for identifying all nutritional problems within any country. Instead, problems are identified from data obtained by either random *ad hoc* surveys or from national nutrition surveys. *Ad hoc* surveys collect data without reference to any systematic scheme for nutritional measurement or any systematic attempt to identify problems. On the other hand, national surveys provide data on the type and extent of nutritonal problems without classifying them or identifying socio-economic causes. Certain areas are over studied or known to be traditionally at risk of malnutrition and are therefore given priority in nutrition planning. Until, for any country, this whole process is systematised, there can be no guarantee of effectively reaching the most nutritionally at risk areas or population groups.

To overcome this we would support any reliable classificatory approach which systematically identifies and classifies nutritional problems. One such system is 'functional classification' which divides any country into primary administrative units, then ecological sub-zones, population sub-groups and then demographic categories which are identified by socio-economic characteristics and types of deficiency problem. This model has not yet been applied but we would support this or any other model providing ecological classifications, community diagnoses or typical profiles of nutritionally at risk areas and groups so long as the approach is systematic and identifies the causes as well as the symptoms of malnutrition.

As part of this new classificatory approach we have tried to identify types of village with specific nutritional problems. We chose to classify nutritional problems at the micro-level in order to identify the whole range of factors responsible for poor nutrition. At this level we can easily identify nutritional problems and their causes and therefore provide meaningful data for the implementation of both curative and preventative programmes. We chose to study problems of *village* nutrition for several reasons. First, because villages are found in most less developed countries and are the primary unit of residence for most rural persons. Second, they are relevant and manageable units for enumeration purposes and therefore form the focus for many studies of rural development problems. Last, the village is primarily a behavioural unit in which most economic, social, political and religious relationships are formed. Villagers live together, eat and work together and share a common cultural heritage, the same values and the same environment.

As an aid to the identification and classification of nutrition problems we have made a collection of village nutrition studies. We feel that these are a sadly neglected but important source of much nutritional information which any planner should use when trying to evaluate and identify problems. Most of the data provided in these studies are of the proximate type providing information on the size and type of nutritional deficiencies but not on their cultural and socio-economic causes and correlates. Data on intra-family distribution of foods and seasonal food consumption are constantly omitted. Individual intakes are rarely measured while average consumption figures are too often expressed in terms of consumption coefficients. Nutrient requirements are hardly ever calculated and intakes are more often compared with standardised recommended allowances. We found that proximate data are rarely analysed in relation to ultimate factors and that nutritional problems of vulnerable groups are analysed independently of their causes. Sadly these gaps made it impossible to conduct a deep and causal analysis of nutrition problems at the micro level.

These findings also have serious implications for the selection and implementation of development programmes. Because we do not have enough information to identify the causes of the problems, policies are limited to alternatives aimed at alleviating the nutrition gap. Either we provide more food through programmes designed to stimulate production or we supplement existing food supplies. But if the real problem is one of poor transportation and inadequate storage facilities instead of limited food supplies, then improving transport systems or providing storage facilities could have more effective results than food supplementation. Similarly, there is little use in making more food available without assessing the effective demand for it. Food availability may be affected by those new inputs but increasing total availability is hardly useful if the disadvantaged sections of the village's population fail to benefit as a result of distributional problems between or within families or over time.

The aims of most of the studies reflect their lack of policy orientation. Although 'primary' objectives had to be deduced from the types of available data, these were far clearer than the 'secondary' aims which should indicate the intended use of the data after collection. General lack of secondary aims indicates that most surveys collect data to measure the size and type of problem but do not evaluate what types of improvement programme would be most relevant to meet needs and cure causes of malnutrition. Similarly, the large base line to resurvey ratio indicates that survey data do not usually provide the basis for any planned action to improve conditions.

There are basically three types of nutrition study conducted at village level: those that provide only nutritional data on food and nutrient consumption, those providing physical measures of nutritional status and lastly, those providing both physical and nutritional data. The majority of surveys provide both types of data. In general, surveys providing only physical data were fewer in number than either food consumption or nutritional status surveys. We found a difference between areas in the types of survey conducted but could find no reliable explanations for this.

We do attempt to interpret the implicit choice of survey type as follows: 'nutritional status' surveys which are very comprehensive and expensive to conduct are formulated in response to vague, unclear, unspecified secondary aims or pure lack of data; 'physical status' surveys, especially those taking only simple anthropometric measurements, provide a quick assessment of the situation and are conducted if resources are limited, while 'food consumption' surveys are conducted to provide quantitative data where nutritional supplementation schemes of one type or another are anticipated. The predominance of nutritional status surveys suggests high costs and the need for different types of information for correct nutritional assessment. Certainly we are finding good evidence from the village surveys that food consumption *alone* does not provide sufficient information because the effects of different food intakes can only be interpreted together with information on disease incidence, work requirements, basic health position and other factors. We suggest that in view of their lack of policy orientation the high cost of most of these surveys cannot be justified. In future, what we suggest is that the alternative ways of measuring nutritional problems must be costed in relation to the accuracy of the data and the needs of planners.

We must evaluate (1) the usefulness and limitations of different types of data for measuring nutritional adequacy in relation to the costs of obtaining it and (2) the costs of obtaining additional information on the causes of malnutrition and the types of ultimate data to collect. Over 2,000 socio-economic studies of single villages have been conducted by social scientists providing a vast data bank of village information and a considerable body of knowledge on how best to go about the collection of socio-economic data. Nutritionists and social scientists should collaborate and combine studies so that nutritionists learn about the collection of socio-economic data and social scientists can be advised on how to collect reliable nutrition data. In this way a considerable amount of additional nutrition data about villages would slowly become available and we may learn more about the causes of poor nutrition.

The initial hypothesis of the Village Studies Programme was that it is the differences among villages that explain the varying success of different sorts of development efforts such that different types of village will respond differently to different types of resource input. Thus a primary aim of the project was to produce a classification of villages by socio-economic variables to form village typologies. Within this framework the aims of the nutrition project were (1) to compare food intakes and requirements in different types of village; (2) to derive estimates of levels of nutrition for villages of different types and to estimate welfare, health and labour quality between villages, and (3) to use evidence from the analyses to estimate the types of village likely to respond best to alternative bundles of measures to improve nutrition. We also feel that the village studies material provides us with unique insights into problems of implementing programmes in villages. By examining (1) village studies of community development, (2) studies which evaluate the impact and problems of programme implementation, and (3) sociological and anthropological accounts of village structure, we realise that introducing nutrition improvement programmes as well as other rural development programmes is not as straightforward as it may at first appear. Unfortunately, most studies evaluating the impact of nutrition programmes measure reductions in nutritional gaps, improvements in nutritional status and reductions in the incidence of deficiency symptoms. Very few measure the success or failure of these programmes in terms of organisational problems, bad project location, wrong approach methods or conflict with village norms and ways of behaviour. In future we would hope that new projects will take note of village political and social structures and will approach individuals, groups and institutions carefully. We should recognise formal and informal power structures, not be too friendly with one faction or group, and be aware of social behaviour, restrictions, belief patterns and group activities. Thus future prescriptions for action will be aware of forces at work within the villages which are both conducive and prohibitive to successful programme implementation.

For both VSP and nutritional purposes, the 'community' aspect of a village was its most essential attribute. Since the village is both a behavioural unit and a rather cohesive entity, we believed that members of the same village would eat the same types, but not necessarily the same amounts of foods and that villages of different types would have different dietary patterns and nutritional problems. Unfortunately our data proved to be rather poor and we were unable to identify enough villages of the same type reliably to formulate village typologies of nutritional problems. Our classification was also based on a non-random selection of village surveys so that although our results are statistically significant, they are not conclusive.

We attempted a classification of village diets by type of main food staple: maize, millet, cassava, potato or rice. This was found to be statistically significant but we were unable to prove that type of main food staple was the key variable responsible for differences between these types of diet. It is possible, for example, that by some coincidence all the cassava villages may have had especially low income levels while all maize villages may have been located near towns.

Similarly we classified village diets by type of village economy; some of our results were significant but again we could not identify economy as the distinguishing variable. Data were too poor to classify village diets by value of food consumption or to test the significance of classifying diets by village location and accessibility. We did, however, find that for a large sample of Indian villages there was a great deal of variation in the total value of cereal and pulse consumption. These values were significantly correlated with average household and *per capita* incomes and with the percentage of families in the village earning less than Rs 750/− per annum; as incomes rise so does the value of cereal and pulse consumption which is also higher in north Indian than south Indian villages. Unfortunately we could not differentiate between home produced and purchased foods but in general, villages purchasing most of their food will be of small land area or have an extremely unequal distribution of land, cash crop villages, villages of agricultural labourers, service villages or perhaps those located near urban conurbations. Village diets are also affected by village location in terms of distance from a town, city or marketing centre and ease of access through communication and transport facilities. These factors could determine both the types of crops cultivated, amounts marketed and types of foodstuffs available to the villagers for purchase. Sale of agricultural produce will affect income levels while village location affects employment opportunities and therefore alternative income sources. All these factors affect the quantities of subsistence foods available, after marketing, for home consumption, the percentage of income spent on food, the amounts and types of food produced and the variety of the diet. Unfortunately, we could test neither the significance of this nor conclude that village location is an important variable.

Although our results are by no means conclusive, they indicate that similar classifications with more and better data based on a random country-by-country sample of village surveys could produce a more reliable typology of rural diets. Our data also indicate that in some villages located in certain ecological and climatic zones not only will nutritional problems differ by type but also by timing. In poorly developed, subsistence villages, where irrigation facilities are non-existent (or at least rain dependent), seasonal climatic changes often dictate the agricultural calendar. This affects, together with other factors, the type, timing and size of crop output. Thus, food consumption levels will vary by season, not only with the familiar factors of seasonal differences in food availability due to harvest timing but also with the effects of other seasonality factors. Seasonal food shortages interlock with seasonality of calorie requirements and of disease incidence. All this affects nutritional status in different ways depending on labour inputs.

Although members of the same village are likely to suffer from the same types of nutritional problem at the same time of year, not all families in nutritionally at-risk villages will be malnourished. Village data are poor but manage to demonstrate the existence of nutritional differences between different income, occupational and religious groups depending on the type of job, the level of resources in the family and dietary restrictions. Not all villages will be alike in these respects; some will be so poor that intra-village differences in income will be negligible; others will be so large that we can identify several groups with different nutritional profiles. These differences have obvious implications for improvement programmes; families may respond differently to the same programme or different groups may need completely different forms of help (education or food supplementation). Unfortunately, villagers are not always able to select what they consider to be relevant programmes so planners must do it for them by evaluating needs and choosing between the alternatives. Specific programmes should be systematically selected to meet specific nutritional problems and needs of at-risk population groups. For (a) any project or team coming fresh into the field or (b) any field-worker wanting a rough measure of how many families are nutritionally at risk or (c) for quick visits by health or food distribution personnel, easy and simple identification of nutritionally at-risk families would save a lot of time and energy. It would mean that preventative and curative medicines could be distributed far more efficiently and fairly, ensuring that only those in need would qualify for help. Thus we have tried to provide some simple guidelines for their identification.

Nutritionally at-risk families include low status, landless, illiterate families of low caste or small *per capita* income who have few resources to meet the nutritional needs of working family members let alone the special needs of vulnerable infants or pregnant women. Children from stable backgrounds will be less at risk than those whose parents have separated or father migrated and failed to send remittances. Family size alone is an important factor creating more competition for food and other family resources for members of vulnerable groups; illiterate, overworked and underweight older mothers are less able to distribute resources fairly and will have less time and energy for child care than younger, healthier, literate mothers.

Village data also indicate that within families certain members are nutritionally more at risk than others. Traditionally we identified pre-school children or pregnant and lactating mothers but we cannot be sure that they are always at risk. We have also identified the mal-distribution of foods as the primary reason for intra-family differences in nutritional status but we really have to examine this in relation to other variables such as disease incidence and size and timing of demands for agricultural labour. Perhaps the whole range of seasonal factors will affect not only the nutritional status of some families more than others but also the nutritional status of certain family members more than others. Our data indicate that in the family food distribution system, priority is usually given to males rather than females. More important is the fact that this includes males of all ages and that sex selective feeding of children is an important variable about which very little is known. More research is needed to find out exactly which members are at risk in which types of family. Unfortunately information is limited and we have primarily identified family types at risk of producing mal-nourished pre-school children rather than any other member. It is most likely that other members of these families will also be at risk but we have no real proof.

We also need more information on why these families are at risk, on what are the causative factors of poor nutrition. We need detailed case studies in order to build up reliable and useful family profiles. These may show that for certain families the best and most economical way to improve nutrition may be to alleviate constraints on female time such as water carrying by introducing pipes or even barrows. But to determine this we need much more detailed information on family activities and on family housekeeping data. We need to know where food comes from at what times of year, who purchases the food, when it is purchased, who decides what food will be bought, how much is stored and what happens when the prices of certain foods rise. We also need more information on economic behaviour, physical activities, type, timing and size of labour inputs of all family members and much more information on the impact of seasonal factors. To put the case more simply, *we need far more micro-level information on nutritional problems and their causes than is available today.*

APPENDIX A: STUDIES OF SEASONALITY IN SELECTED VILLAGES

Table A1: Seasonal Cycle in a Siamese Rice Village in Central Thailand 1953—4

	May[a]	June	July	August	Sept.	Oct.	Nov.	Dec.	Jan.	Feb.	March	April
Season	←———————— Hot, Wet ————————→					←—— Cool, Dry ——→			←———— Hot, Dry ————→			
Temp. (°C)	30	29	28	29	29	28	26	25	25	28	30	30
Rainfall		←— Heavy	Mod.	Heavy —→		←—— Light ——→		←————— Negligible —————→				
Canals		←—— Rising —→			←————— High —————→				←— Lowering fast —→		←— Low , Dry —→	
					High water caused flooding in earth floored cottages							
Travel		←————————— Boat —————————→								←—Travel on foot. Boat travel is difficult because subsidiary canals are dry—→		
Rice cultivation	Plough, harrow and raise seedlings		Heavy transplanting		←— Growing —→		Earliest rice varieties mature	←— Harvest —→				
								Farmers race against the all-too-fast lowering of the water in the canals, without which sheaves could not be moved and buyers could not come for the paddy				
Fruit/ vegetable cultivation	←—— Planting ——→							←————— Annuals die —————→				

Table A1 — *continued*

	May	June	July	August	Sept.	Oct.	Nov.	Dec.	Jan.	Feb.	March	April
Fish supplies	Fish is preserved		Fish available in canals		Fishing is continuous with some preserving			Many varieties of fish mature and men fish night after night				
Labour inputs	Everyone is in the field at dawn		Solid work from dawn-to-dark. Co-operative work and hiring out. Older children work in fields while younger ones (8–13) and the aged look after child care, fishing, cooking and food and fodder gathering		Time for relaxing, visiting, travelling and marketing. Houses and equipment are repaired and the threshing floor is prepared			The villagers worked all daylight hours in the fields and threshed far into the night				
School	Reopens		Vacation					Vacation			Vacation	
Food supplies					Rice in short supply						With time to drain ponds and to fish intensively, people did not need to buy fish and meat which were expensive	

———— Fish and vegetables available in canal ————

Table A1 — *continued*

	May	June	July	August	Sept.	Oct.	Nov.	Dec.	Jan.	Feb.	March	April
Cash availability		Rice sold at this time gets a good price	Debts from capital investments, gambling or ceremonies		←——— Cash jobs ———→			←——— Main rice sale ———→ (Venders are generous with credit but can only navigate the larger canals and are therefore not available to many.)			←— Cash in hand —→	
							←———— Cash is short ————→					
Cash outlay on food			Heaviest cash outlay for family food in transplanting season[b]					Convenience of purchased food is greatest but cash is exhausted			Cash went for capital investments, not food	
Average cash expenditure for meals/day (Bahts)	←——————— 3.93 ———————→				←———— 3.53 ————→			←———— 2.5 ————→			1.53	
Food consumption		Rice consumed in larger amounts. High consumption of green leafy vegetables						Rice consumed in larger amounts			Greater consumption of fish	
Nutrient[c] intake												
Calories			2084			1658			1954		1785	
Protein, g			56			46.5			53.5		61	
Calcium, mg			241			132			154		112	

Table A1 — *continued*

	May	June	July	August	Sept.	Oct.	Nov.	Dec.	Jan.	Feb.	March	April
Iron, mg	←		8.3	→		6.7			9			6.35 —
Vitamin A, i.u.	←		2875	→		1260			1245		1343 —	
Thiamine, mg	←		0.84	→		0.6			0.65			0.6 —
Riboflavin, mg	←		0.54	→		0.25			0.3			0.24 —
Niacin, mg	←		13.6	→		10.1			10.45			11.5 —
Vitamin C, mg	←		31.5	→		32			21			16.5 —

Source: Hauck, H. M. *et al.* (1958), *Food Habits and Nutrient Intakes in a Siamese Rice Village. Studies in Bang Chan, 1952–1954,* Cornell Thailand Project, Interim Report Series No. 4, Data Paper No. 29 (South East Asia Program, Department of Far Eastern Studies, Cornell University, Ithaca, New York).

Notes:
[a] The year starts with May, the beginning of the planting season.
[b] This is 'because of long hours of work, venders again accessible because of high water, cash from sale of last year's crop still in hand, the convenience of cooked foods and snacks, and perhaps the need to replenish household supplies after the long drought, or after their depletion by a ceremony' (Hauck, 1958, p. 13).
[c] These figures were calculated from the mean intakes of two groups of households ($n = 11$). There are no data on seasonal differences in nutrient requirements.

Table A2: Seasonal Cycle in Two Senegalese Villages

	Jan.	Feb.	Mar.	April	May	June	July	Aug.	Sept.	Oct.	Nov.	Dec.
Season					← Wet →							
Crop cycle									← Harvest millet →			
Labour inputs						← Farm work →						
Food supply		← Food abundant →				← Food shortages →						
		← Tomatoes →										

Percentage fulfillment of nutrient requirements in Kour Assane — Fall

	Feb.–Mar.	May–June	Aug.–Sept.
Calories	102	90	73
Protein	86	88	67
Calcium	72	91	67
Iron	136	173	142
Vitamin A	38	44	70
Thiamine	89	92	72
Riboflavin	37	42	26
Niacin	86	90	80
Vitamin C	110	235	58

Percentage fulfillment of nutrient requirements in Sinou Macoumba

	Feb.–Mar.	May–June	Aug.–Sept.
Calories	90	89	73
Protein	93	89	63
Calcium	91	94	96
Iron	115	198	195
Vitamin A	80	140	128
Thiamine	85	98	71
Riboflavin	34	41	26
Niacin	100	109	62
Vitamin C	97	169	80

Source: Hellegouarch, R. et al., *Enquête de consommation alimentaire dans deux villages du Senegal a 3 periodes de l'année.* mimeo (Dakar, Orana).

Table A3: Seasonal Cycle in a South Indian Agricultural Village[a]

	Jan.	Feb.	Mar.	April	May	June	July	Aug.	Sept.	Oct.	Nov.	Dec.
		1			2			3			4	
Season	◄── Cold ──►		◄────── Hot ──────►			◄── Rainy, warm ──►			◄── Wet ──►		
Harvest		Red gram	◄── Vegetables ──►								Groundnuts / Sugarcane / ◄── Rice ──►	
Maximum consumption of food types		Rice / Red gram ◄──── Vegetables ────►			Ragi			Cholam ◄──── Green leaf vegetables (grow along field edges after the rains) ────►			Rice / Groundnuts	
Daily nutrient intake per caput												
Calories		1858			1576			1727			1726	
Protein (g)		44			34			36			41	
Calcium (mg)		586			709			638			540	
Iron (mg)		17.7			16.6			19.9			17.4	
Vitamin A (i.u.)		496			481			784			635	
Thiamine (mg)		1.7			1.7			1.7			1.7	
Riboflavin (mg)		0.6			0.4			0.7			0.7	
Niacin (mg)		18.2			12.7			11.9			14.6	
Vitamin C (mg)		26.7			19.8			36.6			25.7	

Source: Rao, B. R. H. *et al.* (1961), 'Nutrition Status Survey of the Rural Population in Sholavaram. Seasonal Dietary Survey', *Indian Journal of Medical Research*, 49 (2), March 1961, pp. 316–29.

Note:

a Sholavaram village, Vellore Taluq, North Arcot District, Tamil Nadu, South India.

Table A4: Seasonal Cycle in a South Indian Agricultural Village with Data on the Seasonal Variation in the Diets of Pre-School Children

	Jan.	Feb.	Mar.	April	May	June	July	Aug.	Sept.	Oct.	Nov.	Dec.
Season		1			2			3			4	
		←—— Cold ——→		←—— Hot ——→			←—— Warm, moist ——→			←—— Wet ——→		
Harvest				←—— Mangoes ——→								
Maximum consumption of food types	←—————— Green leafy vegetables ——————→											
Nutrient intakes of weaned pre-school children												
Calories		837			1032			753			885	
Protein (g)		18.2			21.8			21.3			24.9	
Calcium (mg)		131			153			135			161	
Iron (mg)		14.4			14.4			11.6			10.8	
Vitamin A (i.u.)		312			323			194			347	
Thiamine (mg)		ND			ND			ND			ND	
Riboflavin (mg)		0.28			0.31			0.35			0.37	
Niacin (mg)		7.6			10.3			6.6			9.8	
Vitamin C (mg)		9.1			13.3			10.9			7.1	

Source: Sundararaj, R. *et al.* (1969), 'Seasonal Variation in the diets of pre-school children in a village (North Arcot District), Part 1; Intake of Calories, Protein and Fat, Part II. Intake of Vitamins and Minerals', *Indian Journal of Medical Research*, 57 (2), February 1969, pp. 249—59; pp. 375—83.

ND = No data.

Table A5: Overleaf

Table A5: Seasonal Cycle in a Forest Village in the Cameroons

	Jan.	Feb.	March	April	May	June	July	August	Sept.	Oct.	Nov.	Dec.
Season				← Wet →				← Wet →				
Crop cycle			Plant maize and ground-nuts	Plant manioc				Plant maize and groundnuts				
Harvest	← Sesame →					← Maize and groundnuts →	← Maize and groundnuts →				Maize and ground-nuts	
Food consumption		Peak fish con-sump-tion	Peak fruit consumption period together with August			Peak consumption of green leafy vegetables		Maximum cereal con-sumption; minimal root/tuber consump-tion; maximum fruit consump-tion Peak vegetable + fish consump-tion				Peak meat consump-tion

———— Period of least cereal consumption ————
———— Period of peak root/tuber consumption ————

Percentage fulfillment of nutrient requirements					
Calories	63	70	61	77	70
Protein	57	60	45	94	94
Calcium	44	27	29	42	20
Iron	81	101	85	80	117
Vitamin A	37	67	71	49	56
Thiamine	70	89	80	152	98
Riboflavin	36	42	43	43	32
Niacin	95	112	86	212	150
Vitamin C	259	396	540	177	295

Source: Masseyeff, R., *et al.* (1958). *Enquêtes sur l'alimentation au Cameroun II. Subdivision de Batouri* (Paris, ORSTOM).

Table A6: Seasonal Cycle in a Forest-Edge, Cash-Crop Village in the South Cameroons

	Jan.	Feb.	March	April	May	June	July	Aug.	Sept.	Oct.	Nov.	Dec.
Season		←— Wet —→			←— Wet —→			←— Wet —→				
Crop cycle			Plant maize + ground-nuts	Plant manioc				Plant maize + groundnuts				
Harvest	←→ Sesame →					←— Maize + groundnuts —→						Maize + ground-nuts
Food consumption			←— Period of maximum food availability —→			Tobacco is sold and the villagers can then afford to buy beef			Period of least consumption, especially of meat, groundnuts and maize		Peak consumption of vegetables + green leafy vegetables ←— Groundnuts —→	
Percentage fulfillment of nutrient requirements in Tikondi village												
Calories	69		73		69		63			46	64	
Protein	62		44		43		72			39	43	
Calcium	34		38		31		25			22	31	
Iron	78		78		77		76			56	76	
Vitamin A	62		37		73		35			31	56	
Thiamine	57		43		73		57			39	46	
Riboflavin	41		34		37		37			31	32	
Niacin	74		62		68		74			60	75	
Vitamin C	453		355		335		240			295	285	

Source: Masseyeff, R., et al. (1958), *Enquêtes sur l'alimentation au Cameroun II. Subdivision de Batouri* (Paris, ORSTOM).

Comments

Table A1

Seasonal differences in food and nutrient consumption are evident in Bang Chan. Calorie intakes vary by as much as 426 calories per head per day and reflect differences in rice consumption. Fortunately calorie intakes are high in the ploughing and planting season but are marginally lower (by 100 calories) at harvest time when energy expenditure is equally, if not more, intensive. Calorie intakes are highest in the period of heaviest cash outlay on family food bought for convenience when the housewife is busy in the fields. At these times, the young children are likely to suffer most as they may be in bed before the main meal of the day is eaten. Consumption of lunchtime meals in the fields could also mean that children miss out at this time too. The convenience of purchased food is greatest at harvest time but this is the period when cash supplies are generally exhausted. However, the maturation of early rice varieties provides useful supplies of rice at times of shortage, just before the main harvest when the villagers worked all daylight hours in the fields and threshed far into the night. Rice shortages are critical at this time but are less critical just before, when the rice is growing and farm work is minimal.

Protein intakes were highest in the period following the harvest because the fish ponds were drained at this time and the villagers had more time to fish intensively. Intakes of Vitamin A were highest from June to August as more green leafy vegetables were consumed although 'better averages of Vitamin A, thiamine, riboflavin and calcium during the first round (June to August) were not such as to provide liberal body stores to be called upon when food supplies of these nutrients were low' (Hauck, 1958, p. 81).

Table A2

In both these villages, groundnuts are the main crop. These are sold for cash but for their consumption the villagers cultivate different varieties of millet. However, there is only one wet season and one harvest of millet. Foods are in shortest supply during the wet season, before new supplies of millet are ready and at the time of heavy farm work. Monetary resources are low at this time of the year and therefore protein intakes are low since the villagers cannot afford to buy meat or fish. Legumes and groundnuts are also in short supply and therefore intakes of thiamine, riboflavin and niacin are low. Consumption of calories and protein is high after the millet harvest.

Table A3

In this village, nutrient intake varied by season, being 'most nearly satisfactory in the first season, less so in the third and fourth seasons and very poor in the second' (Rao, 1961, p. 328). For most nutrients, maximum intakes are achieved in the harvest period of their main food sources: calories in the first and fourth seasons when paddy and pulses are harvested and available at moderate costs; calcium in the second and third seasons when ragi is cultivated; Vitamin A in the last two seasons when green leafy vegetables are abundant; niacin when rice and groundnuts are harvested; and riboflavin when cholam and groundnuts are harvested. There is considerable seasonal variation in the consumption of Vitamin C but intakes are least when green edible leaves are least abundant.

Table A4

It is interesting to compare the seasonal data from A3 and A4 as these two villages are located in the same district of Tamil Nadu. One survey provides data on the diets of pre-school children and the other provides mean per caput data. The pre-school children are fully weaned and consume an adult diet. However, the calorie intakes of the pre-school children are highest (second season) when per caput intakes are lowest. This season is the ragi harvest and fermented ragi gruel is a food commonly fed to the children throughout the year, so they may be provided with extra at this time. Cereals are the main protein source for pre-school children and protein intakes are lowest just after the rice harvest which again suggests they are not fed enough of this food. Intakes are highest in the season of groundnut harvest when children eat raw groundnuts.

Table A5

There is less seasonal variation in calorie intakes in this Cameroon village than in the other villages from India and Thailand. There are several reasons for this: first, there are two rainy seasons which means that two crops of maize and groundnuts can be cultivated. Although only one manioc crop is grown, this, once mature, can remain in the ground until required. The diet is mixed, containing both cereals and roots/tubers which are substituted for each other at different periods of the year. At times of maximum cereal consumption (after the first maize harvest), few roots and tubers are consumed. Their consumption is at a maximum (October, February–June) at times of low cereal intake. There is more inter-seasonal variation in the levels of protein intake; these are lowest in Bokindja village at the end of the first wet season since roots/tubers are the main, but poor, protein source. Seasonal variation in the consumption of other nutrients is also apparent.

Table A6

Tikondi village is subject to a bimodal rainy season; there are two harvests of maize and groundnuts. Although a root crop is also planted, the period of least food consumption is at the end of the second wet season, before the second harvest of maize and groundnuts. Intakes of all nutrients except Vitamin C are lowest at this time of year. Although groundnuts are a good source of protein, maximum protein consumption occurs in July when the cash crop (tobacco) is sold and the villagers can afford to buy beef.

APPENDIX B: CALCULATION OF CALORIE REQUIRE-MENTS FOR TWO HYPOTHETICAL VILLAGES

The characteristics of our reference village and of our two other hypothetical villages are given in the following table:

Table B1: Characteristics of Three Hypothetical Villages

Variable	Reference Village		Village A		Village B	
Population	1000		1000		1000	
Male/female ratio	500 males 500 females		750 males 250 females		250 males 750 females	
Population structure	35% pop. under 20 years 65% pop. over 20 years		30% pop. under 20 years 70% pop. over 20 years		50% pop. under 20 years 50% pop. over 20 years	
Birth and death rates	Medium birth rates Medium death rates Intermediate pop.		Low birth rates Low death rates Old population		High birth rates High death rates Young population	
Population distribution per cent (nos. in brackets)	Male	Female	Male	Female	Male	Female
0– 1 yr.			1 (15)	1 (5)	2.5 (12)	2.5 (39)
2– 3 yr.			3 (46)	3 (15)	4 (19)	4 (63)
4– 6 yr.			2.5 (38)	2.5 (12)	4 (19)	4 (63)
7– 9 yr.			2.5 (38)	2.5 (12)	4 (19)	4 (63)
10–12 yr.			4 (61)	3 (15)	6 (29)	5 (79)
13–19 yr.			2 (31)	3 (15)	5 (24)	5 (79)
20–29 yr.	50 (500)	50 (500)	8 (123)	8 (39)	9 (43)	9 (142)
30–39 yr.			6 (92)	5 (24)	7 (33)	6 (95)
40–49 yr.			7 (107)	7 (34)	5 (24)	4 (63)
50–59 yr.			5 (77)	6 (29)	3 (14)	2 (32)
60–69 yr.			4 (61)	5 (25)	1 (5)	1 (16)
70+			4 (61)	5 (25)	2 (9)	1 (16)
Total	50 (500)	50 (500)	49 750	51 250	62.5 250	47.5 750
Weights of adults (20 yrs+)	Males 65 kg Females 55 kg		Males 80 kg Females 70 kg		Males 50 kg Females 40 kg	
Climate	10°C		−5°C		30°C	
Activity of of males	8 h at 2.5 cal.min. 8 h non-occupational		3 h at 2.5 cal.min. 5 h at 7.5 cal.min. 8 h non-occupational		3 h at 2.5 cal.min. 5 h at 5 cal.min. 8 h non-occupational	
Activity of females	8 h at 1.83 cal.min. 8 h non-occupational		4 h domestic at 3.5 cal.min. 4 h agric. at 5 cal.min. 4 h at 1.41 cal.min. 4 h at 1.83 cal.min.		3 h domestic at 3.5 cal.min. 5 h agric. at 5 cal.min. 4 h at 1.4 cal.min. 4 h at 1.83 cal.min.	

The number of Lusk co-efficients* and the gross total requirements per head were then calculated per village. The results are as follows:

Table B2: Calculated Lusk Values and Gross Total Requirements per Head per Village

	Reference Village	Village A	Village B
Male Lusk population	500	669	201
Gross total required per head	3200	$\dfrac{669}{750} \times 3200$	$\dfrac{201}{250} \times 3200$
		2854	2573
Female Lusk population	350	168	486
Gross total required per head	2300	$\dfrac{168}{250} \times 2300$	$\dfrac{486}{750} \times 2300$
		1546	1490

* The following Lusk co-efficients were used:

Age Group	Co-efficient
Adult male	1
Adult female	0.7
Adolescent (13–19 yrs)	1.0
10–12 yrs	0.8
7– 9 yrs	0.7
4– 6 yrs	0.5
1– 3 yrs	0.4
0– 1 yr	0.3

Net total requirements were then calculated separately for males and females taking age, weight, climate and activity into account. These calculations are as follows:

Table B3: Calculation of the Net Requirements for the Male Population Only

Variable	Reference Village	Village A	Village B
Adult age 20–70 at reference body weight and temperature per cent	100 (3200)	−10% (2885)	−6% (2996)
Adult weight at reference age and temperature	100 (3200)	+17 (3773)	−17 (2644)
Climate on adult requirements at reference age and body weight	100 (3200)	+4.5 (3344)	−10% (2880)
Activity	100 (3200)	+31% (4200)	+8% (3450)
Gross total required per head	3200	2854	2573
Net total required per head	3200	2854 (0.90) (1.17) (1.045) (1.31) 4114	2573 (0.94) (0.83) (0.90) (1.08) 1951

Table B4: Calculation of the Net Requirements for the Female Population Only

Variable	Reference Village	Village A	Village B
Adult age 20–70 at reference body weight and temperature	100 (2300)	−11% (2043)	−5% (2178)
Adult weight at reference age and body temperature	100 (2300)	+20% (2750)	−21% (1824)
Climate on adult requirements at reference age and body weight	100 (2300)	+4.5% (2404)	−10% (2070)
Activity		+23% (2818)	+30% (2998)
Gross total required per head	2300	1546	1490
Net total required per head	2300	1546 (0.89) (1.20) (1.04) (1.23) 2122	1490 (0.95) (0.79) (0.90) (1.30) 1308

The total net calorie requirements caput were then calculated:

Reference Village $= \dfrac{(3200 \times 500) + (2300 \times 500)}{1000}$

$= 2750\ (100\%)$

Village A $= \dfrac{(4114 \times 750) + (2122 \times 250)}{1000}$

$= 3616\ (+31\%)$

Village B $= \dfrac{(1951 \times 250) + (1308 \times 750)}{1000}$

$= 1469\ (-47\%)$

The results show that village A requires 31 per cent more calories per head per day than the reference village while village B requires 47 per cent less. In real life, such extremes will be rare but the variation will be enormous and indicates that requirements should always be calculated for the surveyed population and fieldworkers should not rely on recommended allowances without making adjustments for all other variables affecting requirements.

REFERENCES

Adams, R. N. (1955), 'A Nutritional Research Program in Guatemala' in B. D. Paul (ed.), *Health, Culture and Community. Case Studies of Public Reactions to Health Programmes* (New York: Russell Sage Foundation), pp. 435–58.

Ahmed, M. J. M. and Van Veen, A. G. (1968), 'A Sociological Approach to a Dietary Survey and Food Habit Study in an Andean Community', *Tropical and Geographical Medicine*, 20, pp. 88–99.

Akhauri, N. (1958), 'Socio-Cultural Barriers to Rural Change in an East Bihar Community', *Eastern Anthropologist*, 11(3–4), pp. 212–19.

American Public Health Association (1960), *Control of Malnutrition in Man* (New York: American Public Health Association).

Antrobus, A. C. K. (1971), 'Child Growth and Related Factors in a Rural Community', *Journal of Tropical Pediatrics*, 17, pp. 187–210.

Applied Nutrition Institute (1966–7), *Report of the Work Done in 1966–67*, M.S. University of Baroda, Mimeo.

Ashworth, A. (1968), 'An Investigation of Very Low Calorie Intakes Reported in Jamaica', *British Journal of Nutrition*, 22(3), pp. 341–55.

Attens, M. G. (1969), 'The Shambala System of Agriculture (Usumbara)' in H. Kraut and H. D. Cremer (eds), *Investigations into Health and Nutrition in East Africa*, IFO-Institut Fur Wirtschafts-forschung München Africa – Studienstelle No. 42 (Munich: Weltforum Verlag), pp. 179–219.

Bailey, F. G. (1969), *The Peasant View of the Bad Life*, Communications Series No. 30, Mimeo (Institute of Development Studies, University of Sussex).

Bailey, K. V. (1961), 'Rural Nutrition Studies in Indonesia. III. Epidemiology of Hunger Oedema in the Cassava Areas', *Tropical and Geographical Medicine*, 13, pp. 289–302.

Bailey, K. V. (1962), 'Rural Nutrition Studies in Indonesia. V. Field Surveys: Procedures and Background', *Tropical and Geographical Medicine*, 14, pp. 1–10.

Bailey, K. V. and Whiteman, J. (1963), 'Dietary Studies in the Chimbu New Guinea Highlands', *Tropical and Geographical Medicine,* 15, pp. 377–88.

Bailey, K. V. (1963b), 'Nutritional Status of East New Guinean Populations', *Tropical and Geographical Medicine,* 15, pp. 389–402.

Bailey, K. V. (1964), 'Synopsis of Rural Nutrition Studies in Indonesia', *Medical Journal of Australia,* 1, pp. 669–79.

Bailey, K. V. (1966), *Final Report of a Pilot Project in Applied Nutrition in Bayambang, Paugasinan, Philippines,* Regional Office for the Western Pacific of the World Health Organization, Manila.

Ballweg, J. A. (1972), 'Family Characteristics and Nutrition Problems of Pre-School Children in Fond-Parisien, Haiti', *Journal of Tropical Pediatrics and Environmental Child Health,* 18(3), pp. 230–43.

Batten, T. R. (195(3)), 'Social Values and Community Development' in P. Ruopp (ed.), *Approaches to Community Development,* pp. 80–6.

Belavady, B. and others (1959), 'Studies on Lactation and Dietary Habits of the Nilgiri Hill Tribes', *Indian Journal of Medical Research,* 47, pp. 221–33.

Bengoa, J. M. and others (1959), 'Some Indicators for a Broad Assessment of the Magnitude of Protein-calorie Malnutrition in Young Children in Population Groups', *American Journal of Clinical Nutrition,* 7, pp. 714–20.

Bengoa, J. M. (1973), 'Significance of Malnutrition and Priorities for Its Prevention', in A. Berg, N. S. Scrimshaw and D. L. Call (eds), *Nutrition, National Development and Planning* (Cambridge, Massachusetts: MIT Press), pp. 103–28.

Benneh, G. (1973), 'Population, Food Production and Nutrition in a Northern Savannah Village of Ghana', *Food and Nutrition in Africa,* No. 12, pp. 34–48.

Bennett, F. J. and Saxton, G. A. (1968), 'Family Structure and Health at Kasangati', *Social Science and Medicine,* 2, pp. 261–82.

Berg, A. and Muscat, R. (1972), 'An Approach to Nutrition Planning', *American Journal of Clinical Nutrition,* 25(9), pp. 939–54.

Berg, A. and Muscat, R. (1973), 'Nutrition Program Planning: An Approach' in A. Berg, N. S. Scrimshaw and D. L. Call (eds), *Nutrition, National Development and Planning* (Cambridge, Massachusetts: MIT Press), pp. 248–74.

Berg, A. (1973b), *The Nutrition Factor. Its Role in National Development* (Washington: The Brookings Institution).

Berreman, G. D. (1970), 'Pahari Culture: Diversity and Change in the Lower Himalayas' in K. Ishwaran (ed.), *Change and Continuity in India's Villages* (New York and London: Columbia University Press), pp. 73–103.

Berreman, G. D. (1972), *Hindus of the Himalayas. Ethnography and Change* (Berkely, Los Angeles: University of California Press).

Béteille, A. (1965), *Caste, Class and Power. Changing Patterns of Stratification in a Tanjore Village* (Berkely and Los Angeles: University of California Press).

Blankhart, D. M. (1971), 'Outline for a Survey of the Feeding and the Nutritional Status of Children under Three Years of Age and their Mothers', *The Journal of Tropical Pediatrics and Environmental Child Health*, 17, pp. 175–86.

Bridgeforth, E. B. (1962), 'Statistics in Clinical Appraisals of Nutritional Status', *American Journal of Clinical Nutrition*, 11, pp. 433–9.

Bulatao-Jayme, J. and others (1966), *Baseline Surveys of the Philippines Applied Nutrition Project. Part II. Dietary,* Regional Office for the Western Pacific, World Health Organization WPR/NUTR/23, Mimeo.

Bulatao-Jayme, J. and others (1968), *The Nutritional Re-Evaluation of the Bayambang Applied Nutrition Project II Dietary Survey,* Regional Office for the Western Pacific, WHO.

Burgess, H. J. L. and Wheeler, E. (1970), *Lower Shire Nutrition Survey. A Report of a Nutritional Status and Dietary Survey Carried out in Ngaba Area April/May 1970,* Ministry of Health, Blantyre, Malawi, Mimeo.

Call, D. L. and Levinson, F. J. (1973), 'A Systematic Approach to Nutrition Intervention Programs' in A. Berg, N. J. Scrimshaw and D. L. Call (eds), *Nutrition, National Development and Planning* (Cambridge, Massachusetts: MIT Press), pp. 165–97.

Carstairs, G. M. (1955), 'Medicine and Faith in Rural Rajasthan' in B. D. Paul (ed.), *Health, Culture and Community. Case Studies of Public Reactions to Health Programmes* (New York: Russell Sage Foundation), pp. 107–35.

Chawdhari, T. P. S. and Sharma, B. M. (1961), 'Female Labour of the Farm Family in Agriculture', *Agricultural Situation in India*, 16 (6).

Cleave, J. H. (1970), *Labour in the Development of African Agriculture: the Evidence from Farm Surveys,* Stanford University, PhD Thesis.

Collazos, C. C. and others (1953), 'Dietary Surveys in Peru. I. San Nicolos, A Cotton Hacienda on the Pacific Coast', *Journal of the American Dietetic Association*, 29, pp. 883–9.

Coller, R. W. (1960), *Barrio Gacao: A Study of Village Ecology and the Schistosomiasis Problem*. University of the Philippines, Community Development Research Council (Study Series No. 9).

Collis, W. R. F. (1962), 'Transverse Survey of Health and Nutrition, Pankshin Division, Northern Nigeria', *West African Medical Journal*, 11 (4), pp. 131–54.

Collis, W. R. F. and others (1962b), 'On the Ecology of Child Health and Nutrition. I. Environment, Population and Resources. II. Dietary and Medical Surveys', *Tropical and Geographical Medicine*, 14 (8), pp. 140–63; pp. 201–29.

Connell, J. and Lipton, M. (1973), *Assessing Village Labour Situations in Developing Countries. A Comparative Study of Aims, Concepts and Methods in Village Surveys Bearing on Labour Utilisation*, Institute of Development Studies, Discussion Paper No. 35.

Connell, J. (1975), *Labour Utilization: an Annotated Bibliography of Village Studies*, Institute of Development Studies.

Connell, J., Dasgupta, B., Laishley, R. and Lipton, M. (1976), *Migration from Rural Areas: the Evidence from Village Studies* (Delhi: Oxford University Press).

Connell, J. and Lipton, M. (1977), *Assessing Village Labour Situations in Developing Countries* (Delhi: Oxford University Press).

Cros, J. (1967), 'Enquête Sondage Sur la Consommation des Lipides Dans Quatre Villages du Senegal', *Bulletin de la Societé Medicale D'Afrique Noire en Langue Français*, 12 (2), pp. 153–76.

Cros, J. (1967b), 'État Nutritionnel de la Population de Trois Villages de la Région de Niayes', *Bulletin de la Societé D'Afrique Medicale Noire en Langue Français*, 12 (2), pp. 212–23.

Danda, A. K. (1966), *Planned Development and Leadership in an Indian Village*, Cornell University, PhD Thesis.

Dasgupta, P. (1971), 'Estimation of Demographic Measures for India 1881–1961 Based on Census Age Distributions', *Population Studies*, 25 (3).

Desai, P. and others (1970), 'Socio-Economic and Cultural Influences on Child Growth in Rural Jamaica', *Journal of Biosocial Science*, 2, pp. 133–43.

Devadas, R. P. and others (1965), 'Diet and Nutrition Survey of a Village Community in South India', *Journal of Nutrition and Dietetics,* 2, pp. 83–7.

Devadas, R. P. and others (1969), 'Impact of a Nutrition Education Programme Conducted on the Basis of Findings of a Diet and Food Consumption Survey in a Small Village Community in South India', *Journal of Nutrition and Dietetics,* 6, pp. 115–21.

Dube, S. C. (1955), *Indian Village* (Routledge).

Dube, S. C. (1955b), 'A Deccan Village' in M. N. Srivinas (ed.) *India's Villages* (Bombay: Asia Publishing House), pp. 202–15.

Dube, S. C. (1958), *India's Changing Villages. Human Factors in Community Development* (London: Routledge and Kegan Paul Ltd).

Dwarakinath, R. (1967), 'Community Development as a Means of Organised Social Change', in T. P. S. Chawdhari (ed.) *Selected Readings on Community Development* (National Institute of Community Development, Hyderabad), pp. 1–19.

Dyson, T. (1974), *Analysis and Adjustment of the 1971 Indian Age Distribution and a Reappraisal of Mortality and Fertility Estimates,* Institute of Development Studies, University of Sussex, Internal Working Paper No. 14, Mimeo.

Ekpo, E. U. (1965), *Growth and Development in Relation to Food Intake in Eastern Nigeria,* University of Dublin, PhD Thesis.

Epstein, T. S. (1967), 'The Data of Economics in Anthropological Analysis', in A. L. Epstein (ed.) *The Craft of Social Anthropology* (London: Social Science Paperbacks), pp. 153–80.

Epstein, T. S. (1973), *South India: Yesterday, Today and Tomorrow. Mysore Villages Revisited* (London: Macmillan).

Fernandez, N. A. and others (1965), 'Nutritional Status of People in Isolated Areas of Puerto Rico. Survey of Barrio Mavilla, Vega Alta, Puerto Rico', *American Journal of Clinical Nutrition,* 17, pp. 305–16.

Fernandez, N. A. and others (1966), 'Nutritional Status of People in Isolated Areas of Puerto Rico. Survey of Barrio Naranjo, Moca, Puerto Rico', *American Journal of Clinical Nutrition,* 19, pp. 269–83.

Fernandez, N. A. and others (1968), 'Nutritional Status of People in Isolated Areas of Puerto Rico. Survey of Barrio Montones 4, Las Piedras', *Journal of the American Dietetic Association,* 53, pp. 119–21.

Ferro-Luzzi, G. (1966), 'Rapid Evaluation of Nutritional Level. A Community-Screening Project', *The American Journal of Clinical Nutrition*, 19, pp. 247–54.

Flores, M. and others (1957), 'Estudios de Hábitos Dietéticos en Poblaciones de Guatemala. IX Santa Caterina Barahona', *Archivos Venezolanos de Nutricion*, 8 (1–2), pp. 57–87.

Flores, M. and others (1962), 'Estudios de Hábitos Dietéticos en Poblaciones de Guatemala. X La Fragua, Departamento de Zacapa', *Publicaciones Científicas del Incap.*, No. 59, pp. 106–16.

Flores, M. and others (1964), 'Annual Patterns of Family and Children's Diets in Three Guatemalan Indian Communities', *British Journal of Nutrition*, 18 (3), pp. 281–95.

Flores, M. and others (1965), 'Estimation of Family and Mothers' Dietary Intake Comparing Two Methods (San Antonio La Paz, Guatemala)', *Tropical Geographical Medicine*, 17, pp. 135–45.

Food and Agricultural Organization of the United Nations (1953), *Maize and Maize Diets. A Nutritional Survey.* FAO Nutritional Studies No. 9 (Rome: FAO).

Food and Agricultural Organization of the United Nations (1954), *Rice and Rice Diets. A Nutritional Survey,* FAO Nutritional Studies No. 1 (Rome: FAO).

Food and Agricultural Organization of the United Nations (1967), *Joint FAO/WHO Expert Committee on Nutrition. Seventh Report,* Nutrition Meetings Report Series No. 42 (Rome: FAO/WHO).

Food and Agricultural Organization of the United Nations (1969), *Calorie Requirements,* Nutritional Studies No. 15 (Rome: FAO).

Food and Agricultural Organization of the United Nations (1970), *Requirements of Ascorbic Acid, Vitamin D, Vitamin B_{12}, Folate and Iron,* Nutrition Meetings Report Series No. 47 (Rome: FAO/WHO).

Forster, G. (n.d.), *A Report on Rural Water Use Characteristics in Geographic Sub Areas of the North East Nzega Study Area.*

Fox, R. H. (1953), *A Study of Energy Expenditure of Africans Engaged in Various Rural Activities,* University of London, PhD Thesis.

Fraser, T. M. (1963), 'Socio-cultural Parameters in Directed Change', *Human Organisation*, 22 (1), pp. 95–104.

Fraser, T. M. (1968), *Culture and Change in India. The Barpali Experiment,* University of Massachusetts Press.

Freedman, M. (1955(5)), *A Report on Some Aspects of Food, Health and Society in Indonesia* (WHO, MH/AS/219.55).

Gamble, D. P. (1952), 'Infant Mortality Rates in Rural Areas in The

Gambia Protectorate', *Journal of Tropical Medicine and Hygiene*, 55, pp. 145–9.

Gerhold, C. (1967), 'Food Habits of the Valley People of Laos', *Journal of the American Dietetic Association*, 50, pp. 493–7.

Ginor, F. (1973), 'Importance of the Nutrition Component in Economic Planning' in A. Berg, N. S. Scrimshaw and D. L. Call (eds), *Nutrition, National Development and Planning* (Cambridge, Massachusetts: MIT Press), pp. 275–81.

Gluckman, M. B. (1949), 'The Village Headman in Central Africa', *Africa*, 19 (2), pp. 89–106.

Gluckman, M. (1967), 'Introduction' in A. L. Epstein (ed.), *Craft of Social Anthropology* (London: Social Science Paperbacks), xi–xx.

Gomez, F. and others (1956), 'Mortality in Second and Third Degree Malnutrition', *Journal of Tropical Pediatrics*, 2, p. 77.

Gopalan, C. and Vijaya Raghavan, K. (1969), *Nutrition Atlas of India* (Hyderabad: National Institute of Nutrition, Indian Council of Medical Research).

Gopalan, C. and others (1971), *Nutritive Value of Indian Foods* (Hyderabad: National Institute of Nutrition, Indian Council of Medical Research).

Gordon, J. E. (1965), 'Causes of Death at Different Ages, by Sex, and by Season, in a Rural Population of the Punjab, 1957–1959: A Field Study', *Indian Journal of Medical Research*, 53 (9), pp. 906–17.

Gough, K. (1955). 'The Social Structure of a Tanjore Village' in M. N. Srinivas (ed.) *India's Villages* (Bombay: Asia Publishing House), pp. 90–102.

Gunasekara, D. B. (1958), 'Nutrition Surveys of Some Rural Areas in Ceylon', *Ceylon Journal of Medical Science*, 9 (3), pp. 107–23.

Guyana Ministry of Health (1971), *National Population Nutrition Survey, Republic of Guyana.*

Hartog, A. P. (1970), *Some Aspects of Food Habits in Pantang (a Farming Community in the Coastal Savannah of Ghana),* Regional Food and Nutrition Commission for Africa, Joint Haswell FAO/WHO/OAO (STRC), Mimeo.

Haswell, M. R. (1953), *Economics of Agriculture in a Savannah Village,* UK Colonial Office, Colonial Research Studies No. 8 (London: HMSO).

Hauck, H. M. and others (1958), *Food Habits and Nutrient Intakes in a Siamese Rice Village. Studies in Bang Chan, 1952–1954,* Cornell Thailand Project, Interim Report Series No. 4, Data Paper No. 29 (Ithaca, New York: Cornell University).

Hauck, H. M. and Sudsaneh, S. (1959), 'Food Intake and Nutritional Status in a Siamese Village', *Journal of the American Dietetic Association,* 35, 1149–57.

Hedayat, H. and others (1969), 'Activities of the Centre for Rural Nutrition, Education and Research, Gorg-Tapeh 1965–1967', *Journal of Tropical Pediatrics and Environmental Child Health,* 15 (7), pp. 125–52.

Hedayat, S. M. (1971), 'Birth Weight in Relation to Economic Status and Certain Maternal Factors Based on an Iranian Sample', *Tropical and Geographical Medicine,* 23 (4), p. 355.

Hipsley, E. H. and Kirk, E. K. (1965), *Studies of Dietary Intake and the Expenditure of Energy by New Guineans,* South Pacific Commission, Technical Paper No. 147.

Hitchcock, N. E. and Oram, N. D. (1967), *Rabia Camp. A Port Moresby Migrant Settlement,* New Guinea Research Bulletin No. 14.

Huenemann, R. L. and Collazos, C. (1954), 'Nutrition and Care of Young Children in Peru. II. San Nicolas, a Cotton Hacienda, and Carquin, a Fishing Village in the Coastal Plain', *Journal of the American Dietetic Association,* 30, pp. 550–69.

Huenemann, R. L. and Collazos, C. (1954b), 'Nutrition and Care of Young Children in Peru. III. Yurimaguas, a Jungle Town', *Journal of the American Dietetic Association,* 30, pp. 1101–9.

Huenemann, R. L. and others (1955), 'Nutrition and Care of Young Children in Peru. IV. Chacan and Vicos, Rural Communities in the Andes', *Journal of the American Dietetic Association,* 31, pp. 1121–33.

Huenemann, R. L. and others (1957), 'A Dietary Survey in the Santa Cruz Area of Bolivia', *American Journal of Tropical Medicine and Hygiene,* 6, pp. 21–31.

Hussain, M. (1969), *Progress Report of the First Phase of Lehtrar Applied Nutrition Project, Feb. 1968–1969* (Directorate of Nutrition Survey and Research, Ministry of Health, Labour, Social Welfare and Family Planning, Government of Pakistan), Mimeo.

Instituto Nacional de la Nutricion (1965), *Encuestas Nutricionales en Mexico,* Instituto Nacional de la Nutricion, Mexico.

Interdepartmental Committee on Nutrition for National Defence (1962), *The Kingdom of Thailand. Nutrition Survey, October– December 1960,* ICNND.

Ishwaran, K. (1966), *Tradition and Economy in Village India* (London: Routledge and Kegan Paul).

Ishwaran, K. (1968), *Shivapur A South Indian Village* (London: Routledge and Kegan Paul).

Ishwaran, K. (1970), 'Internal Dynamics of Change in a Mysore Village' in K. Ishwaran (ed.), *Change and Continuity in India's Villages* (New York and London: Columbia University Press), pp. 165–95.

Ishwaran, K. (1970b), 'Introduction' in K. Ishwaran (ed.), *Change and Continuity in India's Villages* (New York and London: Columbia University Press), pp. 1–19.

Jelliffe, D. B. (1966), *The Assessment of the Nutritional Status of the Community*, WHO Monograph Series No. 53.

Jelliffe, E. F. and Jelliffe, D. B. (1969), 'The Arm Circumference as a Public Health Index of Protein-Calorie Malnutrition of Early Childhood. (1) Background', *The Journal of Tropical Pediatrics*, 15, pp. 253–60.

Jelliffe, D. B. (1972), 'Malnutrition in its Total Setting' in B. Vahlquist (ed.), *Nutrition, A Priority for African Development* (Stockholm: The Dag Hammarskjold Foundation), pp. 62–6.

Jelliffe, D. B. and Jelliffe, E. F. (1972b), 'Nutrition and Public Health Planning' in B. Vahlquist (ed.), *Nutrition, A Priority for African Development* (Stockholm: The Dag Hammarskjold Foundation), pp. 126–33.

Jelliffe, D. B. (1972c), 'Nutrition Programs for Preschool Children', *American Journal of Clinical Nutrition*, 25 (6), pp. 595–605.

Jelliffe, D. B. (1972d), 'The At-Risk Concept and Young Child Nutrition Programmes', *Journal of Tropical Pediatrics*, 10, pp. 82–5.

Joy, L. (1972), *Report of Missions to Assist in Food and Nutrition Planning in Iran 1971–2*, FAO, Mimeo.

Joy, L. (1973), in A. Berg, N. S. Scrimshaw and D. L. Call (eds), *Discussion in Nutrition, National Development and Planning* (Cambridge, Massachusetts: MIT Press), p. 239.

Joy, L. (197(3)b), *Food and Nutrition Planning*, Reprints No. 107 (Institute of Development Studies, University of Sussex).

Joy, L. (1973c), 'Nutrition Intervention Programs: Identification and Selection' in A. Berg, N. S. Scrimshaw and D. L. Call (eds), *Nutrition, National Development and Planning* (Cambridge, Massachusetts: MIT Press), pp. 198–206.

Jul, M. (1973), 'Importance of Project Preparation and Evaluation' in A. Berg, N. S. Scrimshaw and D. L. Call (eds), *Nutrition, National Development and Planning* (Cambridge, Massachusetts: MIT Press), pp. 210–12.

Jyothi, K. K. (1963), 'A Study of the Socio-Economic Diet and Nutritional Status of a Rural Community near Hyderabad', *Tropical and Geographical Medicine*, 15, pp. 403–10.

Khare, R. S. (1963), 'Folk Medicine in a North Indian Village', *Human Organisation*, 22 (1), pp. 36–40.

Khare, R. S. (1964), 'A Study of Social Resistance to Sanitation Programmes in Rural India', *Eastern Anthropologist*, 17 (2), pp. 86–94.

King, M. H. and others (1972), *Nutrition For Developing Countries With Special Reference to the Maize, Cassava and Millet Areas of Africa* (Nairobi: Oxford University Press).

Knutsson, K. E. (1972), 'Malnutrition and the Community' in B. Vahlquist (ed.), *Nutrition, A Priority for African Development* (Stockholm: The Dag Hammarskjold Foundation), pp. 46–61.

Knutsson, K. E. (1973), 'Malnutrition: Macrolevels and Microlevels' in A. Berg, N. S. Scrimshaw and D. L. Call (eds), *Nutrition, National Development and Planning* (Cambridge, Massachusetts: MIT Press), pp. 29–33.

Krishnamurthy, (197(4)), 'A Life Cycle. An Anthropological Study of Food Habits' in *Tamil Nadu Nutrition Project Field Reports*, Volume II, Section B, Cultural Anthropology and Nutrition, US AID/Mission to India Report (Haverford, Pennsylvania: Sidney M. Canton Associates Inc.), pp. 30–71.

Lambert, C. M. (ed.) (1976), *Village Studies. Data Analysis and Bibliography*, Vol. 1, India 1950–1975, compiled by M. Moore, C. M. Lambert and J. Connell (Bowker/IDS, London and Brighton).

Lambert, C. M. (ed.) (1978), *Village Studies. Data Analysis and Bibliography*, Vol. 2, Africa, Middle East and North Africa, Asia (excluding India), Pacific Islands, Latin America, West Indies and the Caribbean 1950–1975, compiled by M. Moore, J. Connell and C. M. Lambert (Mansell/IDS, London and Brighton).

Lawson, R. M. (1957), 'The Nutritional Status of a Rural Community on the Lower Volta, Gold Coast', *Journal of the West African Science Association*, 3 (1), pp. 123–9.

Learmonth, A. T. A. (1962), *Sample Villages in Mysore State, India*, University of Liverpool, Department of Geography, Research Paper, No. 1.

Lewis, O. (1954), *Group Dynamics in a North Indian Village*, Programme Evaluation Organisation, Publication No. 1 (Planning Commission, Government of India).

Lewis, O. (1955), 'Medicine and Politics in a Mexican Village' in B. O.

Paul (ed.), *Health, Culture and Community. Case Studies of Public Reactions to Health Programmes* (New York: Russell Sage Foundation), pp. 403–34.

Levinson, F. J. (1972), *The Morinda Experience. An Economic Analysis of the Determinants of Malnutrition Among Young Children in Rural India,* Cornell University, PhD Thesis.

Lipton, M. (1968), *Research into the Economics of Food Storage in Less Developed Countries: Prospects for a Contribution from UK Technical Assistance,* Institute of Development Studies, Communication Paper No. 61.

Madhaven, S. and Swaminathan, M. C. (1966), 'A Comparative Study of Two methods of Diet Survey', *Indian Journal of Medical Research,* 54 (5), pp. 480–5.

Mandelbaum, D. G. (1955), 'Social Organisation and Planned Culture Change in India' in M. N. Srinivas (ed.), *India's Villages* (Bombay: Asia Publishing House), pp. 15–20.

Marriott, M. (1955), 'Western Medicine in a Village of Northern India' in B. D. Paul (ed.), *Health, Culture and Community. Case Studies of Public Reactions to Health Programmes* (New York: Russell Sage Foundation), pp. 239–68.

Marriott, M. (1955b), 'Social Structure and Change in a UP Village' in M. N. Srinivas (ed.), *India's Villages* (Bombay: Asia Publishing House), pp. 106–21.

Marsden, P. D. (1964), 'The Sukuta Project. A Longitudinal Study of Health in Gambian Children from Birth to 18 Months of Age', *Transactions of the Royal Society of Tropical Medicine and Hygiene,* 58 (6), pp. 455–83.

Marsden, P. D. and Marsden, S. A. (1965), 'A Pattern of Weight Gain in Gambian Babies During the First Eighteen Months of Life', *Journal of Tropical Pediatrics,* 10, pp. 89–99.

Martin, W. J. and others (1964), 'Intervals Between Births in a Nigerian Village', *Journal of Tropical Pediatrics and Environmental Child Health,* 10, pp. 82–5.

Maseyeff, R. and others (1959), *Enquête sur L'Alimentation au Cameroun: III Golompoui (Subdivision de Yagoua),* Institut de Recherches Scientifiques du Cameroun, Mimeo.

May, J. M. and Mclellan, D. L. (1973), *The Ecology of Malnutrition in the Caribbean* (New York: Hafner).

Mayer, A. C. (1956), 'Development Projects in an Indian Village', *Pacific Affairs,* 29 (1), pp. 37–45.

McCrae, J. E. (1966), *The Ecology of Malnutrition in a Buganda Village, Uganda,* London University MSc Thesis.

McGregor, I. A. (1964), 'Measles and Child Mortality in the Gambia', *West African Medical Journal,* 13 (6), pp. 251–7.

McGregor, I. A. (1968), 'The Growth of Young Children in a Gambian Village', *Transactions of the Royal Society of Tropical Medicine and Hygiene,* 62 (3), pp. 341–52.

McKay, D. A. and Wade, T. L. (1970), 'Nutrition, Environment and Health in the Iban Longhouse', *South East Asian Journal of Tropical Medicine and Public Health,* 1, pp. 68–78.

Mead, M. (1962), in A. Burgess and R. F. A. Dean (eds), *Malnutrition and Food Habits: Report of an International and Inter-Professional Conference* (London: Tavistock).

Mellor, J. W. (1973), 'Nutrition and Economic Growth' in A. Berg, N. S. Scrimshaw and D. L. Call (eds), *Nutrition, National Development and Planning* (Cambridge, Massachusetts: MIT Press), pp. 70–3.

Mencher, J. P. (1970), 'A Tamil Village: Changing Socio-economic Structure in Madras State' in K. Ishwaran (ed.), *Change and Continuity in India's Villages* (New York and London: Columbia University Press), pp. 197–218.

Mhango, R. (1970), 'Dodoma All Set for a Fresh Start', *Tanzanian Standard,* 17 December.

Miller, E. J. (1955), 'Village Structure in North Kerala, in M. N. Srinivas (ed.), *India's Villages* (Bombay: Asia Publishing House), pp. 42–55.

Ministère des Affairs Économiques et du Plan (1966), *Le Niveau de Vie des Populations de la Zone Cacaoyère du Centre Cameroun,* Societé D'Études Pour la Developpement Économique et Sociale, Paris.

Ministère de la Cooperation, République du Congo (1967), *Quinze Ans de Travaux et de Recherches Dans Les Pays du Niari,* ORSTOM.

Minz, B. (1969), *Impact of Community Development on an Indian Village in the District of Ranchi (Bihar, India). A Study of Planned Social and Cultural Change,* Fordham University, PhD. Thesis.

Moffatt, M. (197(4)), 'Two Anthropological Studies' in *Tamil Nadu Nutrition Project Field Reports,* Volume II, Section B, Cultural Anthropology and Nutrition, US AID/Mission to India Report (Haverford, Pennsylvania: Sidney M. Cantor Associates Inc.), pp. 110–223.

Moore, M. and Lipton, M. (1972), *The Methodology of Village Studies in Less Developed Countries,* IDS Discussion Paper No. 10. (University of Sussex, Institute of Development Studies).

Morley, D. and others (1968), 'Factors Influencing the Growth and Nutritional Status of Infants and Young Children in a Nigerian Village', *Transactions of the Royal Society of Tropical Medicine and Hygiene,* 62 (2), pp. 164–95.

Nair, K. S. (1961), 'Consumption Patterns in Some South Indian Villages', *AICC Economic Review,* June, pp. 15–19.

Newell, W. H. (1955), 'Goshen: A Gaddi Village in the Himalayas', in M. N. Srinivas (ed.), *India's Villages* (Bombay: Asia Publishing House), pp. 56–67.

Nicol, B. M. (1956), 'The Nutrition of Nigerian Children, With Particular Reference to their Energy Requirements', *British Journal of Nutrition,* 10, pp. 181–97.

Nicol, B. M. (1959), 'The Calorie Requirements of Nigerian Peasant Farmers; The Protein Requirements of Nigerian Peasant Farmers', *British Journal of Nutrition,* 13 (3), pp. 293–306; pp. 306–18.

Nietschmann, B. (1972), 'Hunting and Fishing Among the Miskito Indians, Eastern Nicaragua', *Human Ecology,* 1 (1), pp. 41–67.

Oberg, K. and Rios, J. A. (1955), 'A Community Improvement Project in Brazil', in B. D. Paul (ed.), *Health, Culture and Community. Case Studies of Public Reactions to Health Programmes* (New York: Russell Sage Foundation), pp. 349–76.

Office of the Registrar General and Census Commissioner (1972), *Pocket Book of Population Statistics* (India, New Delhi).

Ojha, G. (1969), 'Change in the Pattern of Diet – A Case Study of Orissa Village', *Agricultural Situation in India,* 23 (10), pp. 1037–43.

O'Loughlin, C. (1972), 'What is the Village? The Relevance of Village Studies in West African Social Research', *The Ghana Social Science Journal,* 2 (1), pp. 19–26.

Oluwasanmi, H. A. and others (1966), *Uboma. A Socio-Economic and Nutritional Survey of a Rural Community in Eastern Nigeria,* D. Stamp and others (eds), The World Land Use Survey, Occasional Papers No. 6 (Geographical Publications Ltd).

Oomen, H. A. P. C. (1958), 'Nutrition and Environment of the Papuan Child', *Tropical and Geographical Medicine,* 10, pp. 337–40.

Padmavati, S. and others (1958), 'Diet Surveys in Delhi (1957)', *Indian Journal of Medical Research,* 46 (6), pp. 834–47.

Pan American Health Organization (1973), *Patterns of Mortality in Childhood. Report of the Inter-American Investigation of Mortality in Childhood* by R. R. Puffer and C. V. Serrano, Scientific Publication No. 262 (Washington: PAHO).

Pasricha, S. (1959), 'An Assessment of Reliability of the Oral Questionnaire Method of Diet Survey as Applied to Indian Communities', *Indian Journal of Medical Research*, 47 (2), pp. 207–13.

Patnaick, N. (1969), *Caste and Social Change. An Anthropological Study in Three Orissa Villages*, National Institute of Community Development, Hyderabad.

Paul, B. D. (1952/3), 'The Rational Bias in The Perception of Cultural Differences', *Economic Development and Cultural Change*, 1, pp. 132–8.

Paul, B. D. (ed. 1955), 'Review of Concepts and Contents' in B. D. Paul (ed.), *Health, Culture and Community. Case Studies of Public Reactions to Health* (New York: Russell Sage Foundation), pp. 459–77.

Payne, P. R. (1973), *Report on a Visit to Libya 29 January– 6 February*, Mimeo.

Périssé, J. (1962), 'L'Alimentation des Populations Rurales du Togo. Niveaux de Consommation, Besoins Nutritionels, Depenses Alimentaires, Recommandations Pour Ameliorer l'Alimentation', *Annales de la Nutrition et de L'Alimentation*, 16 (6), pp. 1–58.

Périssé, J. (1968), 'The Nutritional Approach in Food Policy Planning', *Nutrition Newsletter*, 6 (1), pp. 30–46.

Petros-Barvazian, A. (1970), 'The Role of Maternal and Child Health Programmes in the Control of Malnutrition' in P. Gyorgy and O. K. Kline (eds), *Malnutrition is a Problem of Ecology* (Basel, Switzerland: S. Karger), pp. 165–79.

Phillips, P. G. (1954), 'The Metabolic Cost of Common West African Agricultural Activities', *Journal of Tropical Medicine and Hygiene*, 57 (1).

Ramananurthy, P. S. V. and Belavady, B. (1966), 'Energy Expenditure and Requirements in Agricultural Labourers', *Indian Journal of Medical Research*, 54 (10), pp. 977–9.

Rao, B. R. H. and Rao, P. S. S. (1958), 'General Health and Nutrition Survey of the Rural Population in Pennathur. Part III. The Quantitative Dietary Survey', *Indian Journal of Medical Science*, 12 (a), pp. 726–30.

Rao, U. K. and Darshan Singh (1970), 'An Evaluation of the Relationship Between Nutritional Status and Anthropometric Measurements', *The American Journal of Clinical Nutrition*, 23 (1), pp. 83–93.

Rao, K. V. and Gopalan, C. (1971), 'Family Size and Nutritional
    Status' in *Proceedings of the First Asian Congress of Nutrition*
    (Hyderabad: National Institute of Nutrition), pp. 339—48.

Read, M. S. (1970), 'Nutrition and Ecology: Crossroads For Research',
    in P. Gyorgy and O. L. Kline (eds), *Malnutrition is a Problem of
    Ecology* (Basel, Switzerland: S. Karger), pp. 202—17.

Reh, E. (1962), *Manual on Household Food Consumption Surveys*,
    Nutritional Studies No. 18 (Rome: FAO).

Reid, L. M. and Gajdusek, D. C. (1969), 'Nutrition in the Kuru Region.
    II. A Nutritional Evaluation of Traditional Fore Diet in Moke Village
    in 1957', *Acta Tropica*, 26 (4), pp. 331—45.

Ritchie, A. S. (1967), *Learning Better Nutrition. A Second Study of
    Approaches and Techniques.* FAO Nutritional Studies No. 20
    (Rome: FAO).

Sai, F. T. (1973), 'Problems in Nutrition Diagnosis and Planning' in
    A. Berg, N. S. Scrimshaw and D. L. Call (eds), *Nutrition, National
    Development and Planning* (Cambridge, Massachusetts: MIT Press),
    pp. 154—8.

Saunders, L. (1954), *Cultural Difference and Medical Care* (New York:
    Russell Sage Foundation).

Schofield, S. M. (1972), *The Methodology of Village Nutrition Studies
    for Less Developed Countries*, Institute of Development Studies,
    University of Sussex, Mimeo.

Schofield, S. M. (1974), 'Village Nutrition in Less Developed Countries:
    the Nutrition Project of the Village Studies Programme', *Institute of
    Development Studies Bulletin*, 5 (4), pp. 13—20.

Schofield, S. M. (1974b), 'Seasonal Factors Affecting Nutrition in
    Different Age Groups and Especially of Pre-School Children',
    Journal of Development Studies, 11 (1), pp. 22—40.

Schofield, S. M. (1975), *Village Nutrition Studies: An Annotated
    Bibliography*, Institute of Development Studies, University of Sussex.

Scrimshaw, N. S. and others (1968), *Interactions of Nutrition and
    Infection*, Monograph Series No. 57 (Geneva: WHO).

Seoane, N. (1971), 'Nutritional Anthropometry in the Identification
    of Malnutrition in Childhood', *Journal of Tropical Pediatrics*, 17 (3),
    p. 98.

Service Especial de Saude Publica (1956), *Survey in Palmares, Brazil*,
    Rio de Janeiro.

Sharman, A. (1970), 'Nutrition and Social Planning', *Journal of
    Development Studies*, 6 (4), p. 77.

Shiloh, A. (1965), 'A Case Study of Disease and Culture in Action: Leprosy Among the Hausa of Northern Nigeria', *Human Organisation,* 24 (2), pp. 140–7.

Singh, R. and others (1971), 'Diet Survey in Village Gauri in Lucknow District Part II', *Annals of the Indian Association of Medical Science,* 7 (3), pp. 201–15.

Srinivas, M. N. (1955), 'Introduction' in M. N. Srinivas (ed.), *India's Villages* (Bombay: Asia Publishing House), pp. 1–14.

Srinivas, M. N. (1955b), 'The Social Structure of a Mysore Village' in M. N. Srinivas (ed.), *India's Villages* (Bombay: Asia Publishing House), pp. 21–35.

Stoeckel, J. and Choudhury, A. K. M. A. (1972), 'Seasonal Variation in Births in Rural East Pakistan', *Journal of Biosocial Science,* 4, pp. 107–16.

Subramanian, S. R. (1964), *Family Budgets of Rural Families in Kadayanallar Block,* Home Science College, Coimbatore, MSc Thesis.

Sukhatme, P. V. (1971), *The Present Pattern of Production and Availability of Foods in Asia,* Institute of Development Studies Communication No. 1.

Sundararaj, R. and others (1969), 'Seasonal Variation in the Diets of Pre-School Children in a Village (North Arcot District). Part I. Intake of Calories, Protein and Fat. Part II. Intake of Vitamins and Minerals', *Indian Journal of Medical Research,* 57 (2), pp. 249–59; pp. 375–83.

Sundararaj, R. (1972), 'A Comparative Study of the Interview-Questionnaire and Weighment Methods', *Indian Journal of Nutrition and Dietetics,* 9 (1), pp. 13–15.

Tan, M. G. and others (1970), *Social and Cultural Aspects of Food Patterns and Food Habits in Five Rural Areas in Indonesia,* National Institute of Economic and Social Research, Lipi and Directorate of Nutrition, Department of Health, Republic of Indonesia, Mimeo.

Tanzania, Central Statistical Bureau (1963), *Village Economic Surveys 1961/62.*

Tanzania National Nutrition Unit (n.d.), *Report of a Dietary Survey in Kisarawe District,* Tanzania Nutrition Committee Report Series 7A.

Taskar, A. D. and others (1967), 'Diet Surveys by Weighment Method a Comparison of Random-Day, Three-Day and Seven-Day Period', *Indian Journal of Medical Research,* 55 (1), pp. 90–5.

Thompson, B. and Rahman, A. K. (1967), 'Infant Feeding and Child Care in a West African Village', *Journal of Tropical Pediatrics,* 13 (3), pp. 124–38.

Thomson, A. M. (1968), 'A Study of Growth and Health of Young Children in Tropical Africa', *Transactions of the Royal Society of Tropical Medicine and Hygiene,* 62 (3), pp. 330–40.

UNICEF (1967), *General Progress Report,* E/ICEF/558.

University of Ibadan, Food Science and Applied Nutrition Unit (1963), *Results of Surveys Carried out in Osegere, Oje and Moor Plantation,* Fellowship Course in Food Science and Applied Nutrition, Mimeo.

University of Ibadan, Food Science and Applied Nutrition Unit (1966), *Report of Nutrition Studies of Mid-Western Nigeria,* Fellowship Course in Food Science and Applied Nutrition, Papers No. 1–12, Mimeo.

University of Ibadan, Food Science and Applied Nutrition Unit (1968), *Report of Nutrition Survey and Applied Nutrition Programme, Abeokuta, 1968,* Fellowship Course in Food Science and Applied Nutrition, Mimeo.

Usha, T. M. (1964), *A Report on the Community Nutrition Project Conducted in Kalappanaickenpalayan village, Coimbatore District,* University of Madras, MSc Thesis.

Van Velsen, J. (1967), 'The Extended-Case Method and Situational Analysis', in A. L. Epstein (ed.), *The Craft of Social Anthropology* (London: Social Science Paperbacks), pp. 129–49.

Watkin, D. (1962), 'Clinical Appraisal of Nutritional Status of Man, Panel Discussion', *American Journal of Clinical Nutrition,* 11, p. 440.

Wellin, E. (1955), 'Water Boiling in a Peruvian Town' in S. D. Paul (ed.), *Health, Culture and Community. Case Studies of Public Reactions to Health Programmes* (New York: Russell Sage Foundation), pp. 71–103.

White, H. S. and others (1954), 'Dietary Surveys in Peru. II. Yurimaguas, A Jungle Town on the Huallaga River', *Journal of the American Dietetic Association,* 30, pp. 856–64.

World Health Organization (1967), *Joint FAO/WHO Expert Committee on Nutrition,* Technical Report Series No. 377 (Geneva:WHO).

World Health Organization (1968), *Nutritional Anaemias.* Technical Report Series No. 405 (Geneva: WHO).

World Health Organization (1971), *Joint FAO/WHO Expert Committee on Nutrition. Eighth Report. Food Fortification; Protein Calorie Malnutrition.* Technical Report Series No. 477 (Geneva: WHO).

World Health Organization (1973), *The Prevention of Blindness,* Technical Report Series No. 518 (Geneva: WHO).

World Health Organization (1974), *World Health Statistics Annual Vol. 1. Statistics and Causes of Death 1971* (Geneva: WHO).

Wray, J. D. and Aguirre, A. (1969), 'Protein-Calorie Malnutrition in Candelaria, Colombia. I. Prevalence; Social and Demographic Causal Factors', *Journal of Tropical Pediatrics,* 15 (3), pp. 76–98.

Yeshwanth, T. S. and Rajagopalan, R. (1964), 'Consumption of Cereals and Shift from Inferior to Superior Cereals: a Case Study', *Khadigramodyog,* June, pp. 639–46.

Young, C. M. and others (1952), 'A Comparison of Dietary Study Methods. I. Dietary History vs 7 Day Record', *Journal of the American Dietetic Association,* 28, pp. 124–8.

Young, C. M. (1952b), 'A Comparison of Dietary Study Methods. II. Dietary History vs 7 Day Record vs 24 Hr. Recall', *Journal of the American Dietetic Association,* 28, pp. 218–21.

Young, K. (1946), *Handbook of Social Psychology* (London: Routledge and Kegan Paul).

INDEX